Never Give Up . . . All Is Well

DAVID W. HIME

WESTBOW
PRESS®
A DIVISION OF THOMAS NELSON
& ZONDERVAN

WestBow Press books may be ordered through booksellers or by contacting:

WestBow Press
A Division of Thomas Nelson & Zondervan
1663 Liberty Drive
Bloomington, IN 47403
www.westbowpress.com
1 (866) 928-1240

Scripture taken from the New King James Version®. Copyright © 1982 by Thomas Nelson. Used by permission. All rights reserved.

ISBN: 978-1-5127-9363-5 (sc)
ISBN: 978-1-5127-9364-2 (e)

Print information available on the last page.

WestBow Press rev. date: 7/18/2017

Contents

Preface

This book is dedicated to the glory of God and to the loving memory of my parents, Harold L. (April 4, 1918-March 9, 2006) and Virginia N. Hime (January 22, 1913-December 4, 1993), whose love and faithful care of me was the driving force, constant inspiration, and lasting compass for my life. I thank God for my parents and my family and especially for my childhood memories which I would not trade for the world even if I could. **Mother's most famous quote still rings in my ears: "David, you may give in when the going gets tough, but you never give up".** That statement has resonated in my mind throughout my lifetime to give me comfort and inspiration. I grew up as an only child in the Atlanta area, and I am so thankful for my Christian upbringing which has taught me to appreciate what I have and to treat others as I want them to treat me. I believe these qualities and Christian values are the result of my parents having survived the Depression years and being faithful to the church and God during their lifetimes. They taught me to trust in and serve the Lord each day with gratitude, and He will provide for us. I am a kind, caring, and compassionate person who also loves animals and dogs. I enjoy doing things for other people, especially those that are less fortunate than me and those who are suffering physically as well as spiritually and emotionally.

What motivated me to write this book was to reveal and tell the world about my conquest and victory over horrific health problems and physical adversity which cover over 5 decades of my lifetime. I want to inspire others who face seemingly insurmountable odds, outrageous misfortune, and overwhelming physical adversity that nothing is impossible with God to perform miracles for those who believe and trust in Him. I have written this book to give an account of my life experiences that has been told to the best of my knowledge and memory. This book includes discussions and observations from the medical community on such subjects as concussions and brain injuries, collapsed lungs and lung disease, back injuries and the effectiveness of prolotherapy treatments and neuromuscular massage therapy, prostate cancer, hernia repair surgery, and depression. **One fact of life holds true for each one of us: Never take your health for granted. Both your life and health are precious gifts from God. They can be taken away from you in a blink of an eye. Pain never makes an appointment.**

I owe such an unpayable debt of gratitude to so many people, but I will do my best to acknowledge their contributions and kindness toward me and my father for such a long period of time:

Dr. C. R. Hill, Pastor, McDonough First United Methodist Church
Karen DeVan, McDonough First United Methodist Church
Roxanne McManus, McDonough First United Methodist Church
Jack Moore, McDonough First United Methodist Church
Betty Moore, McDonough First United Methodist Church
Jimmie Gorham, McDonough First United Methodist Church
Mary Gorham, McDonough First United Methodist Church
Horace Rowan, McDonough First United Methodist Church
Lib Rowan, McDonough First United Methodist Church
Raford Chambers, Stockbridge Masonic Lodge# 691
Brian Chambers, Stockbridge Masonic Lodge# 691
Marilyn Peskin-Kaufman, Senior Resource Consulting
Mandy Merkel, Senior Resource Consulting
Pastor Landa Larson, Christ the King Lutheran Church
Pastor Sherry Morrison, Christ the King Lutheran Church
Pastor Dave Koppel, Christ the King Lutheran Church
Pastor John Weber, Christ the King Lutheran Church
Ruth Harrivel, Christ the King Lutheran Church
Don Harrivel, Christ the King Lutheran Church
Joyce Crum, Christ the King Lutheran Church
Ray Crum, Christ the King Lutheran Church
Glenn McGuffin, Christ the King Lutheran Church
Susie McGuffin, Christ the King Lutheran Church
Ted Marcis, Christ the King Lutheran Church
John Rhodes, Christ the King Lutheran Church
Lynn Yearous, Christ the King Lutheran Church

Jennifer Fischer, Christ the King Lutheran Church
Bill Jensen, Christ the King Lutheran Church
Lavonne Hallberg, Christ the King Lutheran Church
Sondra Einig, Christ the King Lutheran Church
Jan Arnson, Christ the King Lutheran Church
Ted Spitler, Christ the King Lutheran Church
Al Gantert, Christ the King Lutheran Church
Bob Manka, Christ the King Lutheran Church
Eve Schultz, Florida Department of Revenue
Ron Lee-Own, Florida Department of Revenue
Joe Reach, Florida Department of Revenue
Sam Blackburn, Florida Department of Revenue
Ken Baker, Florida Department of Revenue
Fran Nowak, Florida Department of Revenue
Cheryl McGriff, Florida Department of Revenue
Steven Bayne, Florida Department of Revenue
Bobby Erkhart, Florida Department of Revenue
Randy Brown, Florida Department of Revenue
Jerold Davis, Florida Department of Revenue
Ehshan Peeroo, Florida Department of Revenue
Tom Presley, Florida Department of Revenue
Dr. Mike Moribaldi, Centennial Chiropractic
Lucille Moribaldi, Centennial Chiropractic

Randy Hess, my cousin, gave me the inspiration for part of the title of this book. He said why don't you add the phrase **All Is Well**. I believe that phrase came from the famous hymn **It Is Well With My Soul** which is an awesome and inspiring hymn written by hymnist Horatio Spafford and composed by Philip Bliss. Spafford was inspired to write this beautiful hymn by tragic events in his life: financial ruin caused by losses due to the Great Chicago Fire in 1871 and the loss of all four of his daughters who drowned in the sinking of the *SS Ville du Havre* while crossing the Atlantic. Only his wife Anna survived the tragedy. When Spafford went to be with his wife, the ship's captain alerted him that his ship was passing near where his daughters had died, and he was inspired to write this famous and stirring hymn. Without knowing the story and the tragic circumstances behind the composition of the lyrics, one might not appreciate how moving the hymn is as a source of hope, comfort, reassurance, and encouragement to the bereaved.

I am not "tooting my own horn" when I include a list of my life achievements here. My medical history precedes it simply because it serves as a backdrop for the events in my long life which made me the person I am today. Bo Jackson once said that "[i]f my past didn't happen the way it did, I wouldn't be enjoying the present". As Paul proclaimed so well so long ago in the Bible, we have to turn our disappointments into appointments. C. S. Lewis said it so well about aging. "You are never too old to set another goal or to dream a new dream."

Never underestimate the will power and resolve of your enemies, but then never underestimate the might and power of God who defeats and subdues your Goliaths, including the satanic attacks on your health and well-being. Faithful, God-fearing generations regenerate into faithful, God-fearing generations that follow them. As the Bible tells us in Galatians, Chapter 6, Verses 6-10 [New King James Version], "⁶ [I]et him who is taught the word share in all good things with him who teaches. ⁷ Do not be deceived, God is not mocked; for whatever a man sows, that he will also reap. ⁸ For he who sows to his flesh will of the flesh reap corruption, but he who sows to the Spirit will of the Spirit reap everlasting life. ⁹ And let us not grow weary while doing good, for in due season we shall reap if we do not lose heart. ¹⁰ Therefore, as we have opportunity, let us do good to all, especially to those who are of the household of faith." Always remember that God's infinite strength constantly works within our words, actions, and writing.

Medical History of David Hime At a Glance

Date of Event	Nature of Injury or Illness	Where I was Living at the time	Medical Diagnosis/ Treatment
1960	Double vision and excruciating headache (injured while playing football on the playground during recess at school)	East Point, GA	Severe brain concussion (first of 4 concussions suffered during my lifetime)
1964	5th metacarpal bone broken in right wrist while working out in the high school gym during physical education class	East Point, GA	Cast placed and worn on the wrist for 6 weeks
3/30/1966	Excruciating chest pain and extreme difficulty in breathing while working out on the tennis court during physical education class	East Point, GA	Spontaneous pneumothorax (95% collapsed left lung); surgery performed at St. Joseph's Hospital in Atlanta, GA to reinflate lung
3/9/1967	Experiencing chest discomfort and inability to breathe deep (symptoms similar to those experienced during the remainder of 1966 following the first lung surgery in March 1966)	East Point, GA	Spontaneous pneumothorax (20% collapsed left lung); reconstructive surgery delayed by the surgeon for scheduling later on after the end of the school year

Date of Event	Nature of Injury or Illness	Where I was Living at the time	Medical Diagnosis/ Treatment
3/16/1967	Experiencing chest discomfort and inability to breathe deep on the right side of my chest after leaving the doctor's office	East Point, GA	Admitted to Piedmont Hospital in Atlanta, GA the next day; spontaneous pneumothorax (40% collapsed right lung); surgery performed to reinflate right lung; decision made by the surgical staff to proceed and perform reconstructive surgery of my left lung to prevent it from collapsing in the future
9/30/1967	Experiencing chest discomfort and inability to breathe deep in left lung (symptoms similar to those experienced during the remainder of 1966 following the first lung surgery in March 1966)	East Point, GA	Went to Piedmont Hospital emergency room for examination and X-rays; diagnosed with first lung infection
9/16/1975	Chronic gastritis, indigestion, and discomfort on the left side of abdomen, beginning in early 1974; condition worsened during the year following hospital treatment at Morton Plant Hospital in Clearwater, FL for acute gastritis and dehydration	Dunedin, FL	Initial diagnosis during 1974 was stomach ulcer, and treatment included the use of antacids and prescription for librax to aid digestion; admitted to Morton Plant Hospital in Clearwater, FL with excruciating pain on the right side of abdomen; emergency surgery performed by Dr. John Snelling who discovered and removed ruptured appendix and a large stone wedged in the rectum (doctors did not expect me to live because of gangrene that had spread all over my abdomen)

Date of Event	Nature of Injury or Illness	Where I was Living at the time	Medical Diagnosis/ Treatment
10/8/1981	Severe brain concussion (4th in lifetime); head, neck, back, and knee injuries and trauma to jaw (TMJ) caused by a head-on collision with a drunk driver (uninsured motorist) in Norcross, GA (2nd trauma to jaw after being kicked in the face during a softball tournament in 1980; suffered 3rd brain concussion)	Lawrenceville, GA	Treated at Piedmont Hospital in Atlanta, GA and released; undergone over 20 surgical procedures and intensive physical therapy to treat lower back and hip injuries suffered in the automobile acccident; undergone surgery for TMJ in January 1993 to correct bite with 2 titanium implants
2/26/1998	Acid reflux disease	Stockbridge, GA	Diagnosed through Upper GI series; treated with medications such as Protonix, Prevacid, Nexium, Aciphex, and Dexilant
5/19/1998	Hiatal hernia	Stockbridge, GA	Diagnosed through endoscopy
5/15/2003	Increasing discomfort and swelling involving the area surrounding the appendectomy site	Roswell, GA	Outpatient laparascopic surgery performed by Dr. Barry McKernan in Canton, GA involving the diagnostic examination of the gall bladder and the removal of the adhesions and scar tissue surrounding the appendectomy site
5/17/2003	Blockage in small bowel and an abscess that had formed in the pelvic area and was caused by a tear in the intestinal wall during the laparascopic surgery performed on 05/15/2003	Roswell, GA	Emergency surgery performed by Dr. Rick Finley at Crawford Long Hospital in Atlanta, GA to save my life by removing the blockage from bowel and a portion of small intestine as well as draining the abscess from the pelvis

Date of Event	Nature of Injury or Illness	Where I was Living at the time	Medical Diagnosis/ Treatment
9/21/2014	Whiplash injury to lower back and neck	Roswell, GA	Minor automobile accident (side swiped by another vehicle who was making an illegal left-hand turn out of a parking lot); surgery performed by Dr. Ken Knott in Marietta, GA on injured right hip and lower back
4/14/2005	Hernia or keloid which had developed around the navel area as a result of the major abdominal surgeries in May 2003	Roswell, GA	Outpatient laparascopic surgery performed by Dr. Rick Finley in Canton, GA
2/6/2008	Ultrasound of the abdomen performed to identify and diagnose the cause of the abdominal pain on the right side which indicated the passing of gallstones	Roswell, GA	Outpatient laparascopic surgery performed by Dr. Matthew Novak in Marietta, GA to remove the gall bladder
5/18/2010	Aggressive prostate cancer discovered after undergoing biopsy performed by Dr. Lewis Kriteman in Roswell, GA	Roswell, GA	Intensive radiation treatments as well as 2 consecutive seed implant surgeries on 08/20/2010 and 08/27/2010
7/12/2010	Mycobacterial (MAC) infection discovered in left lung after undergoing bronchoscopy performed by Dr. Dan Callahan in Roswell, GA	Roswell, GA	Treated with multiple antibiotics over a 2-year period
10/31/2013	Increasing discomfort and pain emanating from inguinal hernias discovered during CT and bone scans performed during June 2010 and are protruding from abdomen	Woodstock, GA	Bilateral hernia repair surgery performed by Dr. Michael O'Reilly at WellStar Kennestone Hospital in Marietta, GA

Date of Event	Nature of Injury or Illness	Where I was Living at the time	Medical Diagnosis/ Treatment
3/10/2015	Enlargement and increasing discomfort emanating from an inguinal hernia on the left side of abdomen which had been previously repaired on 10/31/2013 by Dr. Michael O'Reilly; diagnosed as recurrence of hernia in the surgical site	Woodstock, GA	Hernia repair surgery performed on the left side of abdomen by Dr. Michael O'Reilly at WellStar Kennestone Hospital in Marietta, GA

Life Achievements

Taking care of my father who suffered with Parkinson's Disease, prostate cancer, and congestive heart failure from May 2001 until March 9, 2006

Philanthropist (donated thousands of dollars in the form of money, personal items, time, and talents to churches and various charities)

Church Activities

    Ushering at church services
    Counting the offering
    Stewardship Committee
    Audit Committee
    Serving meals at the Wednesday night dinners
    Played church league softball with the following churches:
        Good Shepherd Lutheran Church, College Park, GA
        St. Paul Lutheran Church, Clearwater, Florida
        Norcross First United Methodist Church, Norcross, GA
        Christ the King Lutheran Church, Peachtree Corners, GA

Atlanta Track Club (track and field official/athlete)

J. M. Tull Metals Company Softball Program

    Saved the program from being terminated by the company in 1977
    Managed softball team from 1977-78 and served as general manager from 1977-1983
    Finished in 2nd Place in 1979 and 1981 in league play
    Tournament sponsor and participation

Oversaw construction of the softball field for both men's and women's teams as well as for employees to use and enjoy

Big Brothers and Big Sisters of America

Randy Jones (1978-83)
Karl Lee Martin (1997-2001)

Master Mason in Free and Accepted Masonry in the Grand Lodge of Georgia (January 1980-Present)

Florida Special Olympics (Tallahassee, Florida 1990-1992)

Kiwanis Club in Tallahassee, Florida

Served as Secretary and also Treasurer from January 1990 through September 1992

Volunteer at MUST Ministries in Marietta, Georgia who operate and maintain homeless shelters and food pantries for the needy as well as provide job placement services for the unemployed (March 2013-Present)

Seniors Helping Seniors in Marietta, Georgia (February 2014-Present)

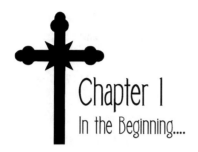

Chapter 1
In the Beginning....

My father's love of music and rhythm was ingrained in me at an early age, so music has inspired and motivated me for decades. An appropriate song entitled **Coming Around Again** performed by Carly Simon contains the lyrics that pretty much set the stage for my life story. A life story that has resulted in one of the greatest comebacks imaginable. My father Harold had urged me to write about my life which, needless to say, has been a journey of faith, courage, and perseverance as well as a testimony to God's grace and faithfulness. I was always so close to my mother Virginia who left me such a legacy of Christian values and moral standards. Her knowledge of the Bible was phenomenal, and it was passed on down to me. She sure was a prayer warrior in the strictest sense of the word. But Daddy knew the Bible, too, and the power of prayer as well. I took care of him the last 4 years of his life as he battled prostate cancer, Parkinson's, and congestive heart failure among other maladies.

My parents came from different backgrounds, but yet they were the same in so many ways. They were both rejected by those they truly loved, and history would repeat itself in my own life later on. Daddy was born on April 4, 1918, the son of a coal miner and carpentry contractor growing up in Minersville, Pennsylvania during the 1920's and the Great Depression. Part of his family emigrated from Germany and came to America to eventually settle in Pennsylvania. Daddy's family was dirt poor, and almost all did not even graduate from high school. I was named after his father, David Benjamin Hime, who had the second most dangerous job in the coal mine—making posts and beams to support and stabilize the mine shafts. My grandmother was Clara Steinheiser Hime whose parents, William and Mary Steinheiser, came from Germany during 1871. Daddy had a brother named Charles and a sister named Anna who passed away at an early age. Tragically for me, both of Daddy's parents passed away during World War II before I was born. As a result, I did not get to know them at all. Ironically, I never got to know my maternal grandparents either. I was told that my paternal grandfather was a "sweet man". Just a few photographs of them here and there are all I have. So far I have not been able to find any evidence of any relatives still living on my father's side of the family. I still have some of my grandfather's tools in the garage—awl, level, hand saws, hand drill, pick ax, and plane for wood carving. And my grandfather's 12 shares of common stock in Miner's Bank which my dad chuckled is not worth the paper it is written on. Well, guess what? At this point in time, the value of this stock is over $6,000 after a 10 for 1 stock split. I think Daddy would have a coronary if he was alive today.

Mysteriously Daddy did not talk much about his family or his past. Apparently it was too painful and sad for him to recall because of the hardships of the Great Depression and the harsh life of growing up in the coal mining region of Pennsylvania. He told me he had the opportunities to go down into the coal mines, but he knew, after his experiences down in the bowels of the mines, that being a coal miner like his father before him was not the kind of livelihood for him. Daddy did enjoy playing "pond" hockey when he was a child. Up north most lakes are frozen over for the bulk of the winter so he must have played hockey a lot.

He always had terrible eyesight and wore thick glasses eventually when his family could afford to buy them. Daddy had to sit close to the blackboard in school so that he could see what the teacher was writing on it. When he was a young boy, he was playing "mumbly peg" with another boy, using a small knife to play the game with. Without warning, the other boy tossed the knife down, and it caromed off the ground and struck my father in the eye. The doctor said that if the knife had hit just a little higher, it would have severed the optic nerve and killed him instantly. My father also talked about the time he and some other boys sneaked underneath the fence at the stadium to watch a football game. He said he would never forget actually seeing Jim Thorpe play in a professional football game in Pottsville, Pennsylvania in the mid-1920's. Just recently I learned that my dad had earned the rank of Star Scout as well as Life Scout in the Boy Scouts. Quite an accomplishment considering his poor and humble beginnings!

Daddy did make it through high school, but later in life he could not afford to attend college on a regular basis to earn a degree in accounting. He tried to go to night school at Georgia State College [University] to get an accounting degree, but he could not manage working for a living full-time and going to school at night. Daddy graduated from Minersville High School on June 12, 1936, the same year Jesse Owens starred in the Berlin Olympics before Adolf Hitler. The start of World War II was brewing in Europe and Asia. To get in the Army, Daddy tried to memorize the eye chart. He did not want to be one of the few men left behind in his town that did not go to war. This attempt did not fool the doctors giving him a physical. They thought he was a "Section 8" trying to pass his physical. Daddy insisted he could serve in the military as a clerk or behind the lines in some capacity. But he did not pass his physicals for the Army, Marines, and the Navy because of his weak eyesight. My dad served his country by working at the Mechanicsburg Naval Depot in Pennsylvania, loading and unloading railroad boxcars for the war effort.

But what is so tragic and distressing to me is that Daddy had loved a lady named Jan during the years before and during the war. Jan had let him know that her mother had passed away at the age of 106, and that was when I became aware of her existence. Daddy began writing letters to Jan 2 years before his death in March 2006. As I understand it, Jan's mother had helped my dad take care of his father who eventually passed away in 1944. They became engaged, and I know my dad was expecting to marry Janet and start a family with her after the war. He told me that he and Jan had had an intimate relationship, and he had already found a house for them to live in. However, for some inexplicable reason, Jan became disenchanted with him, and she decided not to marry him. Instead, she met and married her future husband after a short courtship. I know this disappointment haunted my dad for the rest of his life. I truly believe it soured his disposition and affected not only his relationship with my mother but also with me growing up. He found it difficult to show me affection. Ironically I would experience this kind of misfortune and heartache in my own relationships during my lifetime. I am unsure whether or not this sadness and disappointment also caused my dad's history of stomach problems and ulcers which constantly plagued his life. But I know my dad did have an emergency appendectomy in 1942, and he had suffered phlebitis in one of his legs during his lengthy recovery. Ironically I would suffer the same fate with a ruptured appendix in September 1975.

After the war Daddy lived and worked in New York City for awhile, and he later worked at a hotel in Mount Washington, New Hampshire. He also worked as a night auditor in Fort Lauderdale where he came into contact with the notorious gangster Meyer Lansky, the "Mob's Accountant". My dad told me about the zoot suits and the Benjamins that the gangsters flashed around like dollar bills for tips. He also told me about the bell hop who was constantly checking the seat cushions in the chairs and sofas in the lobby for loose change. Daddy got the opportunity to go and visit Havana, Cuba. It is unknown whether or not Lansky had anything to do with arranging this trip in light of the fact that Lansky was heavily involved in the casinos and organized crime activity on the island at that time.

It was said that my father was blessed with perfect pitch. He had such a great love for music, especially that of the Big Band era—Glenn Miller, Benny Goodman, Tommy Dorsey, Harry James, Vaughn Monroe, Artie Shaw, Gene Krupa, Buddy Rich, and Woody Herman to name a few. His nickname Woody came from Herman. He told me that he and three other fellows went to a Lionel Hampton concert one night, and they were the only white boys in the crowd. My dad loved to play the accordion and had a trombone. I still have the huge collection of "78"phonograph records that are so thick that you can knock somebody out in the head with them. This collection also includes classical music—Bach, Beethoven, Brahms, Chopin, Mozart, Rachmaninoff, Schubert, Tchaikovsky, and Wagner. Daddy also enjoyed George Gershwin and loved the music of world-renowned organist Diane Bish. I know that I inherited my love for music from him. Mother talked about my "happy foot" whenever I was listening to music as a child. Daddy's favorite rock group is the *Bee Gees*. He thoroughly enjoyed watching the 1997 *Bee Gees* live concert twice on PBS before he passed away. My dad also enjoyed the music of *Journey, Elton John, Fleetwood Mac, Beach Boys, Chicago, John Denver,* and *James Taylor.* He was quite intrigued with the unusual voice of Stevie Nicks.

Daddy literally had nothing when he moved to Atlanta in 1948, much less his own car. He had a full-time job as a lowly bookkeeper at Ekonomie Binder Company just to take care of me and Mother. Before he was married, Daddy was mugged in an alley and suffered a severe neck injury that would plague him the rest of his life. A man attacked him from behind with a karate chop. Daddy had no idea what triggered this man's reaction. Doctors said that if the blow would have been any higher, it would have killed him. Daddy began his life-long dependency upon chiropractic care for over 55 years to treat his injured neck as well as stomach problems and other ailments. He must be given credit for his famous remark: **"Pain never makes an appointment"**. I owe a debt of gratitude to Dr. Mike Moribaldi who took such great care of my dad in the last years of his life, even including some "house calls". He came to the house on the last day of Daddy's life. Thank you, Dr. Mike, for your kindness and devotion! You will never be forgotten, my friend.

During his lifetime Daddy enjoyed the outdoors, working on home improvements, gardening, music, model trains, sailing, sports, jogging, and working out at the gym. Starting in 1968 we jogged and worked out together at the gym. During the 1960's my dad became a rabid football fan of Fran Tarkenton and the Georgia Bulldogs. He became an avid sailor with me in 1972. He also managed the softball team during his employment with Fulton Supply Company. Daddy's spirituality and love for God was reflected in his service to the Lutheran and Methodist churches for over 40 years as an usher, offering counter, and capital stewardship committee member. He was a member of Christ the King Lutheran Church in Norcross, Georgia since February 2002 until he passed away. My dad became a Master Mason in January 1980 and is a member in good standing with the Grand Lodge of Georgia Stockbridge Lodge# 691. His dry wit, sense of humor, and compassion for others touched many lives, and his devotion to his family will always be remembered and cherished.

My beloved Mother was born on January 22, 1913 and was raised in Atlanta, Georgia. Georgia State University's first year of existence was 1913. She grew up at 3131 Piedmont Road in Buckhead before it became the fashionable and ritzy *Buckhead* that we know today. Mother was a shy, reserved, and sensitive person who was a devout Christian and loved her family so much. Daddy described her as a Victorian Southern Belle. She was a member of the Nelson family, and she had 2 sisters, Emily Bean and Ann Abigail. The Nelson family is direct descendants of Henry Samson, a 17 year-old passenger on the *Mayflower,* John Alden at Plymouth Rock, and a signer of the *Magna Carta*. This knowledge makes me proud and truly appreciative of the movie *Plymouth Adventure* (1952) starring Spencer Tracy and Gene Tierney. This movie depicts the treacherous journey of the passengers on the *Mayflower* across the Atlantic Ocean. Our ancestors had made their mark and lasting legacy in carving out and forging a new life and existence in what became the Commonwealth of Massachusetts colony.

William Thomas Nelson, my maternal grandfather, was a good, hard-working gentleman who was born on September 6, 1875 and raised in Charleston, South Carolina. My middle name William comes from him. Mrs. Nelson, my maternal grandmother, was born in Forsyth, Georgia on September 6, 1874, exactly the same birthday as Mr. Nelson but a year apart. His father was Samuel Austin Nelson, my great grandfather, who was born in Upton, Massachusetts on October 9, 1819 and one of the direct descendants of a *Mayflower* passenger. He migrated to Charleston when he was 18 years old, and he spent the remainder of his life there. Samuel Nelson eventually joined the Cumberland Church which was destroyed by fire during December 1861.

After the fire, he joined Trinity Methodist Episcopal Church in Charleston where he was a member of that congregation until his death on June 26, 1887. My great grandfather was described by his church congregation as a "…meek, humble, self-denying and, like his Master, he went about doing good. His pecuniary contributions to the Church, the poor, and to all benevolent objects were liberal; and often his friends thought that he gave beyond his means. A favorite remark of his was, '**A Christian man ought to give till he feels it**'." No wonder our family has such a rich heritage and legacy of being so charitable and generous to others over the years.

Another remarkable relative was Ada Hightower (September 11, 1872-April 3, 1963) who was my great aunt on my mother's side of the family. Her nickname was Tippy, and she was hard of hearing. Tippy may have been small in stature, but she was feisty and mighty in the spirit of the Lord. Tippy was such a sweet lady, but you did not dare be fooled by her demeanor because she had a rare and dauntless spirit. I always looked forward to her visits with us because she loved me so dearly. I still have the letters she wrote to me as a child. I guess Tippy's claim to fame is her friendship with a man by the name of John Pemberton who developed the formula for Coca-Cola. She later turned down the opportunity to purchase any common stock in Coca-Cola, citing that the formula contained the now infamous drug cocaine. Of course, the formula was changed to remove the drug from the beverage, and the rest is history. Instead, Tippy invested in an oil and gas lease with Lloyd Oil Corporation of Texas and purchased worthless shares of common stock from Leonard Oil Development Company, B-R Ranch Royalties, Tintic Treasure Mining Company, Pacific States Mines, Inc., Black Gold Petroleum Company, and The Bonanza Gold Mines Corporation. Unfortunately, all of these companies are out of business and defunct. Just think. If Tippy had purchased just 1 share of Coca-Cola common stock in 1919, it would be worth $10 million today! If she had the resources we have today in terms of stock brokers, financial analysts, and endless financial information on the Internet, I truly believe she would have made much better choices and decisions with her investments. Timing is everything in life.

One of the great tragedies of Tippy's life involves her son John Wesley Hightower (1903-August 26, 1964) who was a writer and author. Among his works John wrote *Pheasant Hunting* (1946) which was published by Alfred A. Knopf. John wrote the following words of acknowledgment and praise in the front page of his book: **"To Mother, who is, after all, directly responsible for this book seeing print. Love, Son"**. At the height of his career he became an editor at *Field & Stream Magazine*. Tragically John became a social drinker during his days with the magazine and eventually turned into an alcoholic. He lost his job with the magazine, his wife and family, and everything he owned. John passed away on my birthday in 1964. Mother told me that she saw Tippy kneeling down on her knees many times to pray for her son, but his fate was sealed due to his alcoholism which had destroyed his liver.

Our most famous family member is Charlton Ogburn, Jr. (March 15, 1911-October 19, 1998) who was born here in Atlanta, Georgia. As discussed in *Wikipedia, the Free Encyclopedia, [January 20, 2017]*, Charlton grew up in Savannah, Georgia and New York City. His father was Charlton Greenwood Ogburn, an attorney, and Dorothy Stevens Ogburn was his mother who was an author herself. Charlton's maternal grandfather George Stevens was a long-time book publisher, writer, and former editor of the *Saturday Review of Literature* published by J. P. Lippincott in 1939. His best known work was *Lincoln's Doctor's Dog and Other Famous Best Sellers*. **Stevens entered Harvard at age 14 and *graduated at age 17***. He began his career in book publishing with Alfred A. Knopf and later worked with such notable publishers as Doubleday & Company, W. W. Norton, and J. P. Lippincott.

Another distinguished relative of Charlton is his uncle William Fielding Ogburn who became a famous sociologist.

Wikipedia, the Free Encyclopedia [January 20, 2017], reveals that Charlton, the grandson of George Stevens, also graduated from Harvard in 1932. He became a renowned journalist and writer of memoirs and non-fiction books. During World War II, Charlton served as the communications officer for military intelligence with *Merrill's Marauders*, and he rose to the rank of captain. His most famous work was **The Marauders** (1959), his personal account of the Burma Campaign in World War II, which was eventually made by Warner Brothers into a motion picture titled **Merrill's Marauders** (1962). *Harper's Magazine* carried Charlton's chronicles as one of its cover stories during 1957 which propelled *Harper & Brothers* to propose funding for Charlton to write a book. After the end of the war, Charlton had returned from overseas to begin a career with the State Department under Presidents Truman and Eisenhower from 1946 through 1957, serving as the policy information officer for Far Eastern affairs. He has been recognized as one of the first officials in the State Department during the Eisenhower administration who totally disagreed with the escalation of American involvement in the Indochina War which would later become the Vietnam conflict. Charlton's stance was proclaimed in the book **The First Vietnam War: Colonial Conflict and Cold War Crisis** (Harvard University Press, 2007) written by Mark Atwood Lawrence and Fredrik Logevall. But the offer tendered by *Harper & Brothers* prompted him to leave a rather esteemed government service to write full-time in 1957.

According to *Wikipedia, the Free Encyclopedia [January 20, 2017]*, his literary career began in 1955 with his fictional work *The White Falcon*, a children's story written and published in the *Saturday Evening Post* and eventually made into a Walt Disney motion picture. Charlton also wrote *The Winter Beach* which tells the story about traveling in a remote northeastern shore and earned him the John Burroughs Medal in 1967. Stewart Udall and Roger Tory Peterson described this literary work as a classic of nature writing. Other notable works include *The Bridge*, a story about a teenage girl and her grandfather who are fighting for survival of their way of life, including overcoming threats from family and severe weather; *Big Caesar*, a tale about a boy's love for an old truck, and *The Gold of the River Sea* which was published in 1966 and garnered an award from the Georgia Writers Association for

Charlton's recount of his travel experiences in Brazil. His book *The Adventure of Birds* was published in 1976. Charlton studied such subjects as history, geology, botany, ornithology, and philosophy. As a result, he wrote *The Forging of Our Continent* which was a book on geology for *American Heritage* magazine, and *The Southern Appalachians: A Wilderness Quest*.

Charlton's claim to fame is forever enshrined in several books and articles addressing the authenticity of Shakespeare's authorship of plays and other literary works. In *Wikipedia, the Free Encyclopedia [January 20, 2017]*, he continued his parents' obsession as reflected in their several books on this subject, including **This Star of England: "William Shakes-speare" Man of the Renaissance (Coward-McCann, 1952)**. Charlton's crowning literary achievement is his well-known book, the **1200-page *The Mysterious William Shakespeare: The Myth and The Reality* (New York: Dodd & Mead, 1984)**. His *Oxfordian theory* asserts that these literary masterpieces of Shakespeare actually belong to Edward de Vere, 17th Earl of Oxford (1550–1604). This book energized the substance of the *Oxfordian theory* and generated magazine articles in *The New Yorker* (1988), *Atlantic Monthly* (1991), and *Harper's Magazine* (1999). The Ogburns have claimed that De Vere took the pen name of "William Shakespeare" to cover up a secret love affair with Queen Elizabeth I. Their assertion was De Vere could only write about Queen Elizabeth by hiding his identity under this assumed name which he apparently borrowed from a "dimwit" named William Shakesper who worked in the theater company at Stratford-on-Avon at the time.

What is sad to say is, as I understand it, Charlton was an atheist despite all his literary achievements and contributions during his lifetime. No funeral was held for him in Beaufort, South Carolina where he was living at the time of his death from respiratory failure in 1998.

The Nelson girls all graduated from Agnes Scott College and wanted to marry boys attending Georgia Tech. But none of them ever did. Ann Abigail [Gail] Nelson (July 3, 1911-June 1, 2002) was a Phi Beta Kappa, worked with Dr. Mason Lowance, who used Gail's fluent German for medical records, and was a school teacher for 40 years. Gail married and raised 2 children, James and William Blain, who are my cousins. Emily Bean Nelson (May 7, 1906-June 12, 1985) married and raised 2 children, Virginia and Hubert Bradley, Jr. who are also my cousins. My father met Mother on a blind date, and she would pick him up for a date in her family car which embarrassed him greatly. I do not know how long they dated before they were married. But what is so mysterious and unbelievable is that my parents married on October 15, 1949. Jan and her husband also married an hour apart on October 15, 1949, the exact same day! Jan has 5 grown children and currently lives in Sumter, South Carolina. She still teaches piano to children.

Mother was always so good, kind, thoughtful, and supportive to me and Daddy, too. She was the best cook in the world, cooking homemade apple pie from scratch, fixing Kool Aid popsicles for the children like me, baking chocolate chip cookies, making homemade fudge and pralines, and whipping up maple syrup for homemade pancakes and waffles. When dinner was ready at 6:00 sharp, Mother would say **"Soup's on"**, **Let's Eat Big Feet"**, **or "Dinner is on the table"**. Supper was always at 6:00 at our house, and you dare not be late. I still remember how hard she worked in the house, especially in the summer months without air conditioning, vacuuming and dusting the house, washing dishes, washing and ironing clothes which were first hung up outside on a clothesline to dry in the sun, and scrubbing floors and bathtubs, all done without one single complaint that I can recall. I still remember Mother down on her hands and knees scrubbing the bathroom floor with sweat dripping down her nose but with a big smile on her face.

Mother was totally selfless, forgiving, nurturing when I was so ill during her lifetime, and so positive and optimistic about life which I can attribute to her deep faith in and devotion to God. I remember some of her famous sayings like **"I am going to knock a knot on your head if you don't stop that"**, **"I'll wash your mouth out with soap if you say that word again"**, **"I'll knock you into the middle of next week if you don't stop it"**, and **"They didn't ask me"** when illogical or plain stupid decisions had been made by public figures or celebrities. Mother had majored in mathematics at Agnes Scott so she had no problem helpin me with algebra and mathematics, and I made an A+ in high school algebra. Later in college I would make A+ in calculus, trigonometry, and my first accounting class. I give my mother full credit for my success in school in these subjects. Mother was a **prayer warrior** who prayed for countless people during her long life, friend or foe because she cared so much about people. She did not particularly care about music like Daddy and I did. But I can still hear her sing to herself *I Hear Music and There's No One There* and sing hymns by heart such as *Amazing Grace, All Glory, Laud, and Honor,* and *This is My Father's World.*

Mother's life ended in tragedy in September 1993 when she fell down the steps in the garage of our Stockbridge, Georgia house during a visit to see me. At the time my parents were still living in Tallahassee, Florida. The fall had shattered her left hip so badly that the surgeons could nothing to save her hip or her life. I can still hear the pop of the impact of Mother falling upon the concrete floor in the garage. What still disturbs me is the fact that I could have prevented her from falling down the steps if I had just reacted in time and raced up the driveway to help her come down them. After Mother's arrival at the emergency room of Henry Medical Center in Stockbridge, Daddy and I beckoned Dr. Joseph Dimon III, considered the best orthopedic surgeon in the Atlanta area, to perform the surgery that was needed to repair the severe hip fracture. She had to be moved to Piedmont Hospital where Dr. Dimon took over her care. Later I learned that Dr. Dimon had passed away on March 24, 2014 after a lengthy battle with Parkinson's Disease that also had claimed Daddy's life 8 years earlier. Dr. Dimon gave us both the grim news that there was nothing he could do to repair the shattered hip joint. All he could say over and over again was to give her as much love as possible. We were so devastated we could hardly think straight. Daddy, who had long since retired, visited Mother every day at the nursing home, and I would take time off from work each day to be there with her. Daddy and I did everything humanly possible to ease her pain and make her as comfortable as possible. Nursing homes are notorious for being understaffed and overcrowded which adversely affects the care and treatment of patients.

On the last day of Mother's life on December 4, 1993, I was able to spend the entire day with her at the nursing home since it was Saturday. Daddy had gone down to our Tallahassee house to begin the process of selling it because of our dire circumstances and Mother's plight. After she had eaten her lunch, Mother was lying in a recliner. Nursing home staff described Mother as being "combative" when they attempted to move her in the bed. She had been in such horrible pain and agony from the pin surgically placed in her left hip. **The sight I saw was unbelievable and is still etched in my memory—Mother was gazing upward to heaven with the biggest smile and angelic glow on her face, waving to her family up there with God. It was an experience which I will never forget as long as I live.**

Later in the evening I was about to leave to go home when Mother called me over to her bedside where she gave me a big hug. At that moment I had the sick feeling I was never going to see her alive again after that moment. **I was in total self-denial that she was going to leave us even though I had prayed this most painful prayer in my life that God would take her home to end her suffering.** Mother implored me not to leave her, but visiting hours at the nursing home were over, and I could not stay any longer. The last words I heard her say to me were **"Please don't leave".** I deeply regret that I did not stay with her longer. At 10:45 PM that night I got the telephone call I had been dreading but nonetheless I was expecting. Mother had been taken to the emergency room at the hospital after suffering cardiac arrest. Moments before the telephone call, I knew Mother had left us. **The pain in my left hip that had been injured in the automobile accident in October 1981 had left me and has never returned.** Later in my life I had the great privilege one day of witnessing a radiant aura of light above the head of Kay which I will never forget as long as I live. The love and compassion I had shown in caring for my mother had deeply touched Kay's heart because she had never had a close caring relationship with her mother and father. On May 8, 1996, I was awakened around 5:30AM by an elliptical angelic glow in my bedroom. I was frightened, but only for the twinkling of an eye, because I then heard a spiritual voice that said it was the spirit of Aunt Emily from heaven. It was 11 years after her death. Why I have had the great honor and blessing of witnessing such events I do not know to this day.

After 24 years with Ekonomie Binder Company as a bookkeeper and office manager, Daddy became the credit manager for Fulton Supply Company in 1972 and worked there until his retirement in June 1983. Mother had been much opposed to him seeking employment elsewhere for the fear of changing jobs so late in life. That year he also underwent successful cataract surgery. Unbeknownst to most people, the movie *Driving Miss Daisy* was filmed on location at Fulton Supply Company during 1989 after Daddy's retirement. I remember visiting his company on a few occasions and going upstairs in the building on the grain elevator you see in the movie. You can surely recognize the front of the building located on Nelson Street in Atlanta that was changed to Werthan Bag & Cotton Mill for the film. What is so intriguing is Daddy's company address is the same as my mother's maiden name, Nelson. Is that a coincidence? I really wonder. *Driving Miss Daisy* won an Academy Award for Best Picture in 1989 and deservedly so. The movie brings back so many memories about growing up as a young boy in the segregated South.

I was born a Virgo on August 26, 1950 at Crawford Long Hospital in Atlanta, Georgia. I do believe that the position of the stars and planets at the time of birth do have a bearing on our lives and future in some significant ways. I grew up as an only child in the East Point and College Park area near the Atlanta Airport. I always wanted a brother or a sister to grow up with, but that never happened. I firmly believe that the absence of a sibling in my daily life made it much more difficult for me to mature and socialize with other children since I had no one my age at home to play and identify with. Later on, at the end of Daddy's life, he told me that he had turned down Mother's desire to have another child. Daddy said he was struggling with ulcers and other health problems at the time, and he was working long hours to support us. He knew that decision obviously had caused a growing rift between him and my mother who was running out of time for child bearing. Mother was 37 years old when she had me so "the clock was ticking" for her to have more children which never happened.

I am thankful for my Christian upbringing which has taught me to appreciate what I have and to treat others as I want them to treat me. I believe these qualities and Christian values are the result of my parents having survived the Depression years and being faithful to the church and God during their turbulent lifetimes. They taught me to trust in and serve the Lord each day with gratitude, and He will provide for us. Mother and Daddy were kind, caring, and compassionate people who also loved animals and dogs. We all get great satisfaction and peace in doing things for other people, especially those that are less fortunate than ourselves. To quote Jacob Riis, the 19th Century Danish immigrant to the United States who became a social reformer and a champion for "the stranger in a strange land", **"your past must connect with your present to create your future"**.

To say the least, I enjoyed being a child even though I was a scrawny kid that barely weighed 140 pounds "soaking wet". I was a living example of a "string bean". I was quiet, shy, bashful, timid, self-conscious, and overly sensitive and did not want to have to defend myself. Apparently I was bullied by other kids for supposively being a "mama's boy". In my early days I seemed to get my feelings hurt so easily over what I now realize was nothing. But, all in all, my childhood sure was fun. That's an understatement. I walked in the woods for hours with my faithful dog Punky, a fox terrier, looking for quail (bobwhites). I developed a great love of birds and animals, and I would bring home turtles, toads, lizards, frogs, tadpoles. Playing with Tonka trucks in the dirt, running electric trains, playing ping pong and pool, lifting weights in the basement of our East Point house where I lived from 1957 through 1973. I built a tree house by myself, and I helped Daddy build a carport for our second automobile. We then constructed a basketball backboard and a hoop on top of the carport. I spent thousands of hours shooting baskets. Daddy and I were avid Duke basketball fans and loved Pete Maravich. I loved to play pickup baseball games, go to the movie theater every weekend. We went to the Fox Theatre on several occasions where we saw *My Fair Lady, Dr. Zhivago, How the West Was Won,* and *Guns of Navarone.* Mother and I would have "rainy day" popcorn when it did rain and Pepsis at 3:00 every afternoon. My friend Dennis Hill got me to try bowling, and I spent countless hours over at the bowling alley owned by the Wallace family on Cleveland Avenue in East Point. We would shoot pool for hours and spend I don't know how much money playing the pinball machines. What a great time to be alive and enjoy life in the 1960's! I thought those days and experiences would never end.

I guess my love of dogs began at birth. I do have a baby picture of me sitting next to a cocker spaniel. Technically, my first dog was Buddy who was a terrier mix and ran away from home shortly after we moved into our new house on Dodson Drive in 1957. I was 7 years old at the time, and Buddy never returned home. Our next dog was a little bundle of joy who Mother decided to name Punky. She was a fox terrier and came to us in 1959 and lived throughout my childhood and into my young adulthood. Punky loved to lie in the sun, and her white fur shined like that of an angel. **Hold the word "dog" up in a mirror, and you will have the answer as to what a dog really is. An angel earning its wings.**

I remember one day that Punky was running alongside me when I was riding my bicycle to the grocery store about 2 miles away from the house. It was summer time, and being a child, I did not realize that the summer heat would make the pavement so hot it was burning the soles of her paws. But what was so remarkable was that Punky had not let it slow her down to keep up with me. I finally realized that Punky was hurting, and I examined her paws. Luckily my bicycle was equipped with a basket, and I remember riding my bike all the way back to the house with Punky in the basket with her bleeding paws. I was so deeply touched by my dear friend's sacrifice that I have never forgotten her devotion to me which never wavered. Punky quickly recovered from her ordeal, and the pads on her paws did eventually heal. This experience would change my outlook on life forever.

Another experience was Punky following me to Dodson Drive Elementary School one day without my knowledge. Mother had apparently let her outside and did not realize Punky had followed me all the way to school. She was quite frantic in trying to figure out where she had disappeared to. But, lo and behold, Punky was waiting for me outside after school in the parking lot right next to my bicycle. I was shocked to see her there. Talk about love and devotion! I also remember when my parents and I went to Panama City Beach one summer with Punky. I thought it would be fun to take Punky down to the beach and put Punky in the water. Bad decision! As soon as Punky hit the water, she jumped out and took off like a bolt of lightning for the highway and the rental house where we were staying. How Punky made it back to the house unscathed we will never know except the good Lord. Who would have thought that Punky would live to be 16 years old? Her spirit visited me upon my fateful return from Florida in November 1975 after a neighbor had found her dead in his backyard in July 1975. Sad to say, we have only 2 pictures of our beloved friend for remembrance, but we still have those unforgettable memories and happy times together.

It took my parents and me 5 years to get over the death of our beloved friend Punky. We then decided to look for another dog on the Memorial Day weekend in 1980, the fateful year before the tragic automobile accident that would change my life forever. We found a newspaper ad containing cockerpoo puppies for sale and adoption. Daddy and I went over to check out the puppies, and the dog owner suggested we pick out a female who they thought had personality and was their favorite. I remember having a hard time keeping the little guy in the box we had to take her back home in. Mother eventually named her Spunky who she said was "a sweet dog in a rough sort of a way". She followed us wherever we went. I had never seen a dog get so much out of life. After relocating to Florida, Spunky loved to go out in the sailboat in the Gulf of Mexico with Daddy and me. When you ever said the word "boat", Spunky would go bonkers and dance in a twirl and knew she was going to have the time of her short life on the boat. She loved to chase Frisbees and tennis balls you threw to her, gnaw on chew toys, and play "rubber tug of war". I remember that both Punky and Spunky loved to lick Eskimo ice cream and popsicle sticks. That was so funny to watch them.

Spunky became ill in early 1987 and was diagnosed with yellow jaundice. On March 29, 1987 I spent the last day with my beloved friend lying in my lap. It was Sunday, and I knew deep down inside that Spunky was not going to survive another day. As she lay in my arms, I was gazing into the dying dog's eyes, and God spoke to me and said to open the Bible on the lamp stand. He then told me to read what I saw which was **First Corinthians, Chapter 15, Verses 50 through 55 [New King James Version]**, which says:

> "⁵⁰ **Now this I say, brethren, that flesh and blood cannot inherit the kingdom of God; nor does corruption inherit incorruption. ⁵¹ Behold, I tell you a mystery: We shall not all sleep, but we shall all be changed— ⁵² in a moment, in the twinkling of an eye, at the last trumpet. For the trumpet will sound, and the dead will be raised incorruptible, and we shall be changed. ⁵³ For this corruptible must put on incorruption, and this mortal *must* put on immortality. ⁵⁴ So when this corruptible has put on incorruption, and this mortal has put on immortality, then shall be brought to pass the saying that is written: "Death is swallowed up in victory. ⁵⁵ O Death, where *is* your sting? O Hades, where *is* your victory?"**

I had never read these scriptures before in my life. **Again, hold the word "dog" up in a mirror, and you will have the answer as to what a dog truly is: God's unconditional love**. When I left the house, I knew it would be the last time I would see Spunky alive as she watched me walk out the front door. The next day Mother called to let me know that Spunky had passed away. They found her lying lifeless between their beds, loyal and loving until the end of her short life on earth.

After the loss of our beloved Spunky, it felt like we all had lost a child, and we were so devastated and consumed with grief. She had lived a mere 7 years. A few months later, my parents began the search for another dog. They found a newspaper ad where the owner of a giant Schnauzer was relocating to Virginia Beach, Virginia and could not take his dog along with him. He wanted to find a good home for her. My parents fell in love with the dog right away and decided to adopt her. I found it difficult to accept this dog after losing Spunky whom we had raised from a puppy and were so close with for such a short period of time. We did not realize that we were beginning a whole new chapter in our lives with our choice and love of Schnauzers. This breed of dog originated in Germany in the 15th and 16th centuries. The term comes from the German word for "snout" because of the dog's distinctively bearded snout. Although the Schnauzer is considered a terrier-type dog, they do not have the typical terrier temperament.

The Schnauzer type consists of three breeds: the giant, standard, and miniature. Toy and teacup are not breeds of Schnauzer, but these common terms are used to market undersized or ill-bred miniature Schnauzers. The original Schnauzer was of the same size as the modern Standard Schnauzer breed and was bred as a rat catcher, yard dog, and guard dog. Friendly and loving, Schnauzers become part of their families and can get along well with children if raised and socialized properly. They are protective and energetic and will alert members of the household to any potential danger. The Schnauzer is always alert and makes an excellent watchdog, although its watchful nature can lead to persistent barking.

Missy was our first Schnauzer, a giant. Her name came from her original owner. For some inexplicable reason, I decided to change her name to Misty after watching *Play Misty for Me* [1971] starring Clint Eastwood, one of our favorite actors, Donna Mills, and Jessica Walter. And the name has stuck with us ever since. Misty I (the first Misty) would stand perfectly still while you groomed her fur. She loved taking a bath, jumping into the bath tub without pleading her to do so. Misty I would come into my bedroom and ask me, "What's on the docket for today, David?". Misty loved going out on the boat and riding in the car. Daddy would say that Misty I would sit in his lap in the car "just like a princess". I used to take Misty I to the nursing home where Mother was, and you could see the faces of the residents light up. Misty I also loved to chase lizards and other critters. She would die of colon cancer in 1998 after spending 11 wonderful years with us. Daddy and I tried to save her life, but the cancer was terminal, and there was nothing that the vet could do. We had to put Misty I down because she was hurting so bad. Daddy told me later that "I will never do that [euthanize] again, David". He was so heartbroken, and so was I.

It was not long before Daddy and I began our search for another dog. We were still grieving over the loss of Mother. In the local newspaper, we saw a picture of a Schnauzer that was available for adoption at the Henry County dog pound which eventually became our second Schnauzer, Misty II. Daddy and I spared and saved her from the dog pound who was about to euthanize her. It was difficult, at least for me, to deviate from the name Misty, and so this dog who was nameless came to be known as Misty II. She was a wild dog about a year and a half old according to the vet that Daddy and I did not realize needed constant supervision and monitoring. I now fondly remember her as Mischief, and she surely lived up to that name. Mischief chewed on furniture, shoes, clothing, socks, even the carpeting in the house. Daddy was so upset he said we might as well take her back to the dog pound where we found her. However, we turned to the vet for advice, and he told us to put her in a crate to calm her down. That did the trick, and this dog like her predecessor became a great and faithful companion and friend to both of us. Mischief loved to play with tennis balls, socks, bedroom slippers. Daddy enjoyed taking her for long walks. When I decided to adopt Buddy, a Cairn terrier, in September 2005 as a companion for Mischief, she loved and enjoyed playing with him so much that they became close. She always enjoyed going out on the sailboat on Jackson Lake before we had to move to Roswell. Later, as my dad said, Mischief became my "buddy" and closest friend when he became so ill and spent so much time in assisted living and hospitals. I could not have survived emotionally without her companionship during this stressful time of adversity and sadness. Mischief went everywhere with me as my constant companion at the assisted living facility, nursing home, and the hospital.

Mischief's exposure to contaminated food and water during her wanderings and in the dog pound probably were the culprits that damaged her liver and eventually caused lymphoma. She passed away at my feet on the hearth of the fireplace on February 16, 2006, exactly 3 weeks before Daddy left us on March 9. I never told him that Mischief had passed away. At that point in time I began looking for another Schnauzer even though I still had Buddy, the Cairn terrier. I used the Internet for starters, and I searched *PetFinder.com* where I found a Schnauzer who was being given up by a young family in Johnson City, Tennessee. Jessica and Ron Christian (that's right Christian) were having a tough time making ends meet trying to take care of their 4 small children. I began communicating with them before Daddy passed away. They told me that 5 other people had inquired about their dog. I eventually told them that my dad had since passed away in the meantime.

I remember the day I went to the cemetery with my dad's ashes. It was March 25, 2006, and on that day I was notified by the family that the dog had been promised to a lady that the dog was hers, and she was going to pick her up that day. I was so disheartened to hear that. When I got home from the cemetery, I had an E-Mail from the couple who told me the lady never showed up to claim their dog. **I will never forget what Jessica said, "God meant for you to have our dog."** I still have a copy of this E-Mail. I sobbed for joy. What is so astounding to me is this dog's name is Misty. I did not give her that name.

During the nine years that Misty was with me, we endured so many hardships, trials, and tribulations after my dad passed away. I had worked for the State of Florida as a sales tax auditor since I was hired in Sarasota, Florida in October 1984. Legal wrangling and disputes over tax law interpretation and application; potential taxpayer confrontations; gathering defensible documentation to support our position in the audit findings; interruption of audit schedules due to the lack of cooperation by taxpayers to produce records for review; difficulty in sleeping in hotel rooms and living "out of a suitcase" on the road; disruption of audit trips by inclement weather, and management's constant monitoring of your completion of audit assignments, this type of work is obviously not for "the faint of heart". A tax auditor has to wear many "hats" in this job—accountant, computer analyst, secretary, writer, Columbo, Perry Mason, negotiator, diplomat, and credit manager. What was so disheartening and insurmountable to me as an auditor was management's evaluation of your audit performance which was predicated upon the resources and cooperation of taxpayer personnel who are never under the control of the auditor at any time.

I had sacrificed my health to take care of Daddy, but the toll it took on my mental, emotional, and physical well-being was devastating and irreversible. I had suffered with a bad gall bladder for many years, and I had to ignore the pain and discomfort to keep going because I was the only one that Daddy had in our small family to take care of him. Eventually my gall bladder was removed on February 6, 2008 by Dr. Matthew Novak after countless trips to Atlanta Gastroenterology during 2007 to treat my symptoms. The surgeon showed me a photograph of my gall bladder which was totally gray in color. Dr. Novak told me that the normal color of a healthy gall bladder is bluish-green. I had lived with a defective gall bladder for nearly 10 years.

Complicating my life even more was my battle with prostate cancer and a mycobacterial lung infection that were simultaneously diagnosed in May and July 2010, respectively. Unbeknownst to most people, I was diagnosed with "aggressive" prostate cancer, and I had to undergo 25 intense radiation therapy treatments, plus 2 back-to-back seed implant surgeries in August 2010. During all these difficulties and suffering was my faithful friend Misty who was always by my side. I was never alone with her there and, of course, with God's presence. I will never forget the prayers of so many people at our church and at the office where I worked. I felt those heart-felt prayers every day which gave me great comfort and encouragement.

In March 2013 Misty was diagnosed with borderline Cushing's Disease which is a terminal illness and attacks the pituitary and adrenal glands. Typical symptoms of this illness are excessive drinking of water and urination, excessive eating, panting, overweight, potbelly, and seizures. Eventually Misty's seizures became more frequent and more intense. In July 2014 the vet put Misty on Phenobarbitol for the seizures which seemed to diminish them. She had been breathing so heavily the last couple of days so I knew something was wrong with her. The vet took X-rays of Misty's abdomen and also her lungs since she felt Misty might have fluid in her lungs. The vet found an enlarged liver and possible tumor which was pressing on her lungs and made it so difficult for Misty to breathe. The tumor had also moved the spleen out of position. The vet felt that exploratory surgery could be done to determine if the tumor could be removed, but she thought Misty may not survive any operation because of her age and deteriorating physical condition. I could have brought Misty home with me, but she would probably have not survived the night and would have passed away in agony at the house. I had to focus on Misty's welfare and quality of life before thinking about my own. But it was still difficult and so disheartening to let her go. I could not stop sobbing at the vet. I felt like I had lost a child. I know Misty is in heaven with Daddy who gave her to me as a gift for taking care of him for such a long time. There is no doubt in my heart about that. That is why I am so sad that she is not here anymore because of her link to

Daddy. I realize now that I had spent so much time in the company of death all these years.

In 1980 Christopher Cross wrote his famous song *Sailing* which described so well the sailing experience and adventure. I have always been fascinated by boats and sailing ships. My home contains countless pictures or paintings of sailboats, a Yankee Clipper, and all types of ships. My dad and I had built, well, assembled our first sailboat in May 1972. He had found a magazine ad where Kool cigarettes were promoting their tobacco products through the sale of Snark sailboats called daysailers. It was approximately 11 feet long, and Daddy and I had to put the fiberglass cloth all over the hull of the sailboat ourselves under the cover of the open carport. I still remember mixing the epoxy resin to glue the cloth on and the strong smell. After reading the instructions for beginners, I learned how to sail on a small pond in Stockbridge for starters and eventually on Stone Mountain Lake. I have a photograph of Daddy fumbling around with the sails and the halyards supporting them. We would transport the sailboat and its mast to the nearest lake on racks fastened to the top of the car, along with the sails, oars, and life vests. Our favorite lakes were Lake Lanier, Lake Hartwell, and later Lake Sinclair near Eatonton, Georgia.

During 1980 Daddy and I decided to look into purchasing a larger sailboat. We found a used Siren 17 for sale at a local dealer. This sailboat was built by Vandestadt & McGruer located in Ontario, Canada and is light-weight and handles extremely well when reaching or tacking into the wind. Also, we were looking for a sailboat with a cuddy or cabin to store our gear, for camping out, and for protection from inclement weather. Daddy and I enjoyed the Siren 17 for so many years and eventually took the boat with us when we resettled in Sarasota, Florida in June 1983. The greatest sailing experiences my dad and I had were out in the Gulf of Mexico. Of course, there were some bad storms out in the Gulf, *no name storms* to be exact, that appeared out of nowhere and tested your sailing skills as well as your resolve and mettle. But I can never forget the sight of pelicans and gulls as well as dolphins swimming alongside the boat. My dad and I made the decision in 1991 to purchase yet another sailboat, the Hunter 18.5 made by Hunter Marine Corporation but now known as Marlow-Hunter LLC located in Alachua, Florida. This sailboat was heavier in weight at 1,400 pounds but was durable and stout in the strong currents in the Gulf with a bulb wing keel designed for the Americas Cup competition.

What is so sad to me is the lack of interest in sailing shown by the women I have dated. Whenever I took a lady out in the sailboat, that was only an uneventful one-time experience for her. One of my friends calls a sailboat a "blow boat". I guess what most people enjoy is being out on a speed boat like a Sea Ray or MasterCraft, pontoon boat, bass boat for fishing, or possibly a houseboat. Any boat that can go faster than a sailboat. I became a Big Brother in October 1978, and Randy Jones and Karl Martin enjoyed going out on the sailboats and also working on them. When I am out on the water, I want to get away from the hustle and bustle of life and, quite frankly, I am in no hurry to go anywhere in particular. It is a great chance to get fresh air out on the water and relax to get away from the stress and strain of life.

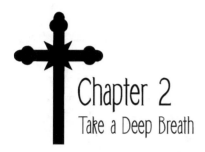

Chapter 2
Take a Deep Breath

January 1966....

East Point, Georgia. Sophomore at Headland High School. The '1960's. President John F. Kennedy had been my hero growing up, but now he was gone. I have come to the realization that the United States of America has never recovered from the assassination of Abraham Lincoln. Then, nearly 100 years later, President John F. Kennedy, my boyhood hero and champion, was gunned down on November 22, 1963. Camelot and the Age of Innocence died with him, and our great country has not been the same since. Just as catastrophic was the Supreme Court decision in the same year prohibiting prayer in the schools. Anti-war protests, Civil Rights marches, the "glory suits" of the Ku Klux Klan, hippies and the psychodelic drug culture, long hair and mini-skirts, bell bottoms, the Beatles, Buffalo Springfield, Elvis Presley, and the Cold War filled the pages of newspapers and *Time* magazine, Huntley & Brinkley, Walter Kronkite, TV shows, and countless Hollywood movies. Anybody over 30 could not be trusted. I had the sad feeling that my childhood was coming to an end, and I had no clue about what life was all about. I was just a wet nose kid and a living example of a "string bean" at 6 foot 2 inches tall and 140 pounds. As I said before, I was shy, bashful, timid, quiet, and sensitive and did not want to have to defend myself. To me it was a sad time in my life as I was approaching 16 and feared growing up. College seemed light years away as far as I was concerned. It was tough for me just to get through high school with flying colors much less think about what I wanted to do with my life. I was so shy and bashful that I couldn't get enough courage to talk to girls, much less ask them out on a date. Carol, my childhood sweetheart, was still in my heart, and I felt so out of place because she was so popular with the student body and, of course, I was not. As I look back at my youth, I now feel I took it for granted that this girl was truly my soul mate for life, and God had placed her in my life for that specific purpose. But being so young I really had no idea what life was all about and the impact of poor choices and bad decisions on my life. There is no doubt in my mind that God always places people in our lives for different purposes or reasons.

I knew one thing though: I was blessed with blazing speed and running ability. During the tryouts for Little League baseball, I had outrun everybody in the sprints. I was beginning to realize that I did indeed have athletic ability which had shown in playing my first year in Little League baseball when I was named an All-Star pitcher. But for me at age 8 athletics did not appeal to me that much. I was so nervous whenever I went out on the baseball field. My self-confidence and self-esteem were just non-existent. Little did I know at the time that my athletic abilities and competitiveness would be sorely tested and play such a pivotal and defining role in my life's journey. One of the greatest mistakes I ever made was dropping out of Little League baseball after only 2 years. Hindsight is always 20-20.

I decided to test my running ability and try out for the track and field team at Headland. The football players were all worshipped as gods it seemed like to me, and a good many of them were track stars, too. Maybe I could generate some female interest in me much less some self-confidence by becoming a "jock". I began to run after school and work out with weights in January 1966. My dad had bought a York barbell set for me for Christmas, and I started to work out at the house on my own. You have to realize at that particular time in the 1960's there were no Bally's, Gold's Gym, LifeTime Fitness, or a neighborhood YMCA nearby. Lifting weights like Jack LaLanne? Jogging? What's that? I was thankful just to have a pair of Keds or baseball cleats which were glued to my feet. I was so proud of those cleats I did not want to take them off. I had a J. C. Higgins baseball glove which I cherished.

I had no clue how to train to run competitively. And I did not see eye to eye with the football and track coach. He could be best described as a master sergeant in cleats and with a whistle and an intimidating disposition like that of Gunnery Sergeant Foley in *An Officer and a Gentleman*. I was literally intimidated not only by the coach but also what seemed to be the impossible task of proving myself and making the team. I was also concerned about my school work that I thought would suffer by trying out for track and field.

Going to college was definitely the next item on my life's agenda, at least where my parents were concerned. I knew that it would take a great deal of time to get stronger physically to compete, something I began to dread again. It seemed like I was always a bundle of nerves or had uncontrollable "nervous energy" that I could not harness. I guess I considered myself a failure right off the bat until I proved otherwise. But ironically running track and jogging was going to be a huge part of my life later on....

March 30, 1966....

8:45AM

The most serious injury or ailment that I had ever suffered up to this point in time was a severe concussion playing, of all things, "touch" football at recess at school when I was 10 years old. I had run back 2 kickoffs for touchdowns, so the other team thought we need to teach this kid a lesson. On the next kickoff, I was "gang tackled" by at least 3 boys who drove my head into the ground. I was helped off the playground because I was so woozy from the collision, and I had double vision and a severe headache afterwards. But I did not fumble the football. I went to school the next day just to show those boys responsible that I was tougher than they were. I still have the bony knot in my forehead where my head hit the ground. It was the first of 4 serious concussions that I have suffered during my lifetime. Daddy told me that this head injury would plague me the rest of my life and cause future health problems. It turned out to be a prophetic statement.

The day started at Headland High School like any other day. My first class after home room was Physical Education or PE as we called it. As usual I dressed out for class, and we were playing tennis that fateful day. I do not remember feeling ill or under the weather before I left for school. It was like any other sunny but cool day in March. I enjoyed playing tennis, and I had great rapport with Coach Short who had respect for me as a young naïve boy just trying to do my best. I had no idea that what was about to happen was going change my life forever. We had just started to play tennis when I began to experience some discomfort in my chest. I told Coach Short that I was not feeling too well, and I needed to sit down to see if the pain would subside and go away. I sat down on the tennis court for a few moments.

However, I was beginning to hurt more and more, and I was noticing I was having problems breathing and catching my breath. I decided to ask Coach Short if I could return to the locker room to change clothes and go home sick. The pain and discomfort in my chest was becoming too much for me to bear, and I staggered all the way to the dressing room. I barely made it to the principal's office, and I called my mother to tell her I needed to come home. I reckon it was about 9:30AM when I called home, and I broke down and began to sob uncontrollably, the piercing pain was so unbearable. I was terrified about the thought of dying right there on the spot.

Daddy immediately came from work to pick me up in his Volkswagen and take me back to the house. Once I got home I tried to lie down, but the pain was so intense I could not relax or find any comfortable spot to relieve the pain. One of my dad's famous quotes was **"pain never makes an appointment"**. What was happening was my left lung was collapsing, and as I tried to lie down, the lung would shift in my chest like a balloon losing air and rub up against my chest cavity. The pain was absolutely indescribable. I was so scared and terrified at what I was experiencing that I thought I was going to die because the pain was so unbelievably excruciating. Taking a deep breath was just about impossible without pain.

My parents decided to rush me to the nearest doctor to see what was going on. In that day and age there were no ambulances much less paramedics on call. Under normal circumstances we would have gone straight to Dr. Mason Lowance, our family doctor, whose office was in downtown Atlanta, but Dr. Cobb's office was closer to the house. I had earlier gone to Dr. Cobb when I had broken my right wrist in 1964. Later Dr. Lowance would tell us he was so disappointed that we did not come to see him. What now seems so ironic is Daddy drove me by himself to Dr. Cobb's office. Daddy and I were not too close when I was growing up. I did not get much support from Daddy when I was considering sports activities. His time was so consumed by having to work long hours, including overtime on Saturdays, and selling the *World Book Encyclopedia* on week nights. As a result, Daddy had little free time to play catch with me or shoot baskets. I can recollect the time when Carol and I were throwing a baseball to each other in the backyard. Carol threw the baseball over my head, and it hit and broke the window pane on the garage door. Mother and I feared Daddy's temper, and we hurriedly went to a glass dealer in town to find a window pane to replace the broken one before Daddy got home from work. After several attempts, we finally got the glass to fit in the window, and Daddy never found out that we had broken it. I always felt that I was to blame, not Carol.

Now I remember the long, tortuous drive to the doctor, especially when we went over the railroad tracks at Lee Street. The pain was so terrible that I thought I was going to pass out or die. Dr. Cobb examined me and took X-rays of my chest and lungs. Without hesitation he determined that my left lung was collapsed 95%, and I must be taken to the nearest hospital immediately for treatment and possible surgery to reinflate my lung. A **collapsed lung or spontaneous pneumothorax** is the gradual accumulation of air in the pleural space between the lung and the chest wall. With the increase in the amount of air in the pleural space, the pressure against the lung causes its collapse. This pressure prevents the lung from expanding properly when you try to inhale, causing shortness of breath and chest pain that is indescribable. A collapsed lung may become life-threatening if the pressure in your chest prevents the lungs from getting enough oxygen into the blood. An injury such as a broken rib or puncture usually causes a collapsed lung, but it may occur suddenly without an injury. Chronic obstructive pulmonary disease (COPD), asthma, cystic fibrosis, and pneumonia can also cause collapsed lungs. Spontaneous pneumothorax can also occur in people who do not have lung disease.

The initial theory was that air-filled blebs or blisters had formed on the top of my lung which had burst and caused the collapse of the lung. What I failed to reveal to the doctors was that I did smoke a few cigarettes in my early teens before trying out for track and field. Running may have caused the formation of these blisters because my lungs were not fully developed for my height. Dr. Cobb referred my case to St. Joseph's Hospital in Atlanta where Daddy and Mother took me to be examined by Dr. Newton Turk IV and Dr. Rodriguez, the attending physicians, thoracic specialists, and surgeons on staff at the hospital.

As I lay in the emergency room, I started to believe that I would never leave this place alive. I was experiencing excruciating pain and lying in a hospital bed propped up did not help at all. It seemed like an eternity until I was taken up to my room which I shared with 3 other patients. Dr. Turk and Dr. Rodriguez came into my room, and they injected me with a shot of Novocaine to supposively numb my chest. I remember that the hypothermic needle the doctors used was at least 5 inches long. The surgeons then proceeded to cut a hole in the left side of my chest near my heart while I watched in utter horror. The doctors placed a long red rubber hose through the incision into my chest cavity, and then they attached the other end of the hose onto a bottle of water on the floor next to my bed. I still remember the surgeons sewing up my incision. Why on earth the doctors did not put me under anesthesia I will never know. I was obviously in no position to argue. I could actually feel this hose inside my chest as I tried to move around on the bed. Eventually the doctors placed a catheter in my bladder to help me urinate because I was literally bed-ridden with no way for me to get up and go to the bathroom. I cannot forget the pain and discomfort of that chest tube and catheter inside me. There I was 15 years old and in a room full of strangers, totally oblivious as to my fate or the prognosis for my recovery. I never felt so helpless and terrified in all my existence.

I lay flat in the bed for 5 straight unbearable days and nights. I tried to watch television to take my mind off myself and my suffering, but I just could not find a comfort zone. My eyes became so blood shot that I could hardly see. I can still hear the hospital intercom blaring out the call for **Dr. Fincher, Dr. Ronald Fincher**. The only time I moved was the time I was taken downstairs to have X-rays taken of my left lung. When I was carried down to the X-ray room, I was left out in the hallway on a gurney waiting for my turn. All of a sudden I looked up, and there was this immaculately dressed woman standing next to me. In an instant I knew I recognized her; it was Coretta Scott King, the wife of Dr. Martin Luther King, Jr. I must point out that this is April 1966. Merely 2 years from this point in time Dr. King would be assassinated in Memphis, Tennessee. What is quite intriguing to me is my dad was born on April 4, the day Dr. King was killed in 1968, Daddy's 50th birthday.

I was so happy that I got a get well card from Carol. **The "girl next door" truly was Carol Hunt.** She was born on March 21, 1950 so she is five months older than I am. We enjoyed playing together, especially Simon Says with our neighbor Judy Reardon, and when we got the rare chance to go to the community swimming pool. I remember her kissing me on the cheek along the way home from school one day. I still remember the spot. I guess we were about 8 years old at the time, and that was my first kiss and last for a long, long time. Carol's father, James Hunt, had decided to keep us from seeing each other for reasons that I or my parents never knew or understood. One day the St. Bernard got loose from the Hunts' fenced in backyard. The dog came running down our driveway, but I was not afraid of him. He decided to put his front paws on my shoulders and look me straight in the eye. We were literally eyeball to eyeball when Mr. Hunt emerged and grabbed the dog by the leash without saying a word. Hello, how are you? Thank you. Nothing. No matter. Those were fun times that I will never forget. Later in 1970, this beautiful girl became Miss Atlanta.

It made me feel good that someone cared about me. I know my parents certainly did during those long days and nights in the hospital where I stayed for 2 weeks. Dennis Hill, my boyhood friend, came by one night to see how I was doing. Emily, my beloved aunt, visited me during the time I was in the hospital. Mother was my constant companion there at my bedside. She was always my "bestest" friend. Both of my parents took such good care of me. Godly people whose faith was being sorely tested for the first time with me and my fate.

After 5 days of suffering as I lay so rigidly in a hospital bed, the doctors decided to remove the awful tube from my chest. When the tube was removed, I yelled at the top of my lungs. At least I tried to. In a few days I was discharged from the hospital, still not knowing what my fate was. When I arrived home after my ordeal at the hospital, my left lung was still not healed. It is extremely difficult to explain how I felt about the condition of my lungs. My left lung was bothering me as I just tried to breathe normally or move around. My chest was so irritated and uncomfortable that I could not relax. From March 30, 1966 until the end of the year, I did not feel well, and my left lung constantly bothered me with discomfort. I did not feel confident about taking chances to be active or be around others. I was definitely feeling despair about my life and what was going to happen in the future. Gloom, fear, and uncertainty seemed to dominate my thinking all the time.

In early March 1967 I suffered my second collapsed left lung after school. I returned to Dr. Turk's office where I again had my left lung X-rayed. Dr. Turk delivered the sad news to Mother and me that my lung was again collapsed but fortunately only 40% this time. He said that I would have to undergo major surgery after school was over in the summer to reconstruct my left lung so that it would not collapse again. Believe or not, my cousin Brad's former wife Marie had suffered collapsed lungs and had had the same type of surgery Dr. Turk was going to perform. As we left the doctor's office, we were in the elevator and going back to the house, and I turned to Mother and I said, "I believe my right lung is starting to collapse". This feeling of losing air in your lungs has never left me. The day was March 16, 1967, and now both my lungs were collapsed, a fatal condition if not treated immediately. My parents called Dr. Turk and let him know what was happening. He contacted Piedmont Hospital who informed us that they did not have any beds available until the next day. I would have to spend the night at home and be admitted to Piedmont Hospital first thing in the morning to confirm my condition and act accordingly.

In the evening I began to actively die as I started vomiting gray matter which is a sign of near death. **I have learned one important fact about this experience: You know when you are going to die. But there are no bells ringing, no drum rolls, no trumpets sounding, no curtain call. You are alive one minute and then gone the next.** At approximately 1:00AM on the morning of March 17, 1967, I died and began to float over my bed. Mother was sleeping by my bedside, but she was unaware of what was going on. I remember feeling the sensation of touching the sky with my hands. I saw my life as I had lived it flash before my eyes in nothing flat. Then there was a white light that appeared out of nowhere, but I noticed it did not hurt my eyes to gaze upon it. I heard the voice of God who spoke telepathically to me, and He did all the "talking" to me. God said that He was giving me a second chance to live because He had a divine plan for my life. God is indeed a God of second, third, fourth….. and a hundred chances. I am living proof of that spiritual reality.

It was much later in my life in July 1988 when I was sitting in a pew at the Oneco First United Methodist Church near my home in Bradenton, Florida when God came to me telepathically and told me to open the hymnal in my lap. Without any hesitation I opened it up, and God said to read the passage I had in front of me. The scripture was in the book of consummation **The Revelation of Jesus Christ, Chapter 21, Verses 22-27 [New King James Version]**:

"**²² But I saw no temple in it, for the Lord God Almighty and the Lamb are its temple. ²³ The city had no need of the sun or of the moon to shine in it, for the glory of God** illuminated it. The Lamb *is* its light. [24] And the nations of those who are saved shall walk in its light, and the kings of the earth bring their glory and honor into it. [25] Its gates shall not be shut at all by day (there shall be no night there). [26] And they shall bring the glory and the honor of the nations into it. [27] But there shall by no means enter it anything that defiles, or causes an abomination or a lie, but only those who are written in the Lamb's Book of Life."

God then revealed to me that this scripture describes what I saw on that fateful morning of March 17, 1967. I still cannot explain how God communicates with me. All I can say is it is mental telepathy or extrasensory perception with the thoughts and images placed in my mind. I can remember getting into the car for the long journey with my parents to Piedmont Hospital after awakening from what I thought was my last breath on earth. This would be the first of other encounters with God who only promises us each day and each breath that we take. I remember the ride to the hospital and a sense of hopelessness which I had felt since this nightmare had begun in March 1966. Here I was 16 years old, and I was preparing myself for the extremely painful surgical procedures to reinflate my right lung with the insertion of the tube in my chest as before as well as major reconstructive surgery on my left lung. The doctors had to reinflate my right lung first before performing the delicate operation to tie my left lung to my chest cavity to prevent further collapsing of that lung in the future.

A few days after my right lung was reinflated, I underwent the reconstructive surgery on my left lung. Dr. Turk had to "jack up" my ribs to enable the surgeons to attach my lung to my rib cage and then remove the top part of my lung in order to take out the blisters causing the lung to collapse. I still have the long wide scar where Dr. Turk opened up my ribs. I owe Dr. Turk, Dr. Rodriguez, and the surgical staff at Piedmont Hospital my life. I remember thick tubes protruding from the side of my chest. I tried to get up during the night after the surgery because I had to go to the bathroom so bad, and I almost passed out and fell flat on the floor. I don't remember how long I was in the hospital. When I eventually returned to school, the doctors recommended to the principal that I carry a reduced course load for the remainder of the school year. I had to go to summer school in June 1967 because I had gotten so far behind in my school work. Summer school was a first for me. **A funny thing about life: it sure finds a way to go on with or without you.**

Even months after the surgery, I would wake up in the middle of the night or first thing in the morning and take a deep breath to see if my lungs had collapsed again during the night. Any ache or pain in my chest made me think immediately that I was having yet another collapsed lung. In fact, in September 1967 my parents rushed me to the hospital because I was experiencing the symptoms of a collapsed lung on my right side. Dr. Rodriguez diagnosed my condition as a lung infection, the first of many during my lifetime. Later in 1968 I actually met a gentleman at the health club where Daddy and I worked out who told us he had suffered 2 collapsed lungs on each side. He showed us the scars from the surgeries. He was a good bit older than me but with the same build and physique as me, tall and lanky.

At that particular time physical therapy was in its infancy, and once the surgeons discharged you as a patient, you were basically on your own for healing and recovery through proper diet and exercise. You were literally "thrown to the wolves" to survive. All I could think of was to start working out slowly with light weights. Here again, I had no one to guide me like a personal trainer or physical therapist. While working out with weights, I may have aggravated my left shoulder which had been apparently damaged during the reconstructive surgery on my left lung. I literally had to learn how to breathe all over again. Logically I reckoned that I would have to first build up my chest and shoulders and then I could improve my breathing and lung capacity. I later would learn how to breathe properly when I was lifting weights, exhaling during the lift of the weights and inhaling as I lowered them.

Because of the lung surgeries that disrupted my life during high school from March 1966 through December 1967, I was totally unprepared to go to college not only mentally but also physically and emotionally. While I was battling for my life, my friends were out having a good time and enjoying life as teenagers. **Life goes on.** No question that my physical adversity and suffering had traumatized both me and my parents because its magnitude had taken such a toll on all of us. I knew I had to focus entirely on finishing my senior year of high school. Unfortunately, I had little or no guidance as to where to go to college or how to channel my interests into a successful career when I got out on my own. I had spent so much time, energy, and effort in enduring pain and agony, recovering from so many surgeries, battling illness and my own self-doubts and fears, overcoming death, and spending the entire summer in school that it was rather anticlimatic in a way when it came to choosing a college or a course of study. I felt I had been deprived of part of my teen years in 1966 and 1967 that I could never recoup or relive. When I graduated from Headland High School on May 15, 1968 with honors, everyone was so excited and joyous about finishing high school. I did not feel such joy since I had 4 more years of schooling at college staring me in the face. I was totally "burnt out" with school and education for that matter. It seemed like I could not rekindle my desire or will to resume my educational pursuits and find my identity in a college or university. I am not sure why I chose Catawba College in Salisbury, North Carolina over schools such as Davidson, Lenior-Rhyne, Elon, Guilford, or any other college. I did not even consider Georgia State, the University of Georgia, or Georgia Tech. Why I do not know. As I look back, I desperately needed serious counseling and aptitude tests to guide me in determining the right course of study and career to help me choose the university or college to attend.

When I arrived at Catawba College in September 1968, classmates in my dormitory taunted and made fun of me when I described the horrors of my collapsed lungs and surgeries. They thought a collapsed lung was so funny and treated me as a wimp. I could not understand or tolerate their lack of compassion and concern for my well-being and the suffering I had endured. I would not wish the excruciating pain of a collapsed lung even on my worst enemies, even these heartless guys who were literally harassing me at every turn it seemed. I began to ask myself, "What am I doing here putting up with this childish behavior and their attempts to humiliate me?" After a brief time, I made the decision to leave Catawba College and return home. I had gone there for the specific purpose of getting a college education to get ahead in life, but these pathetic jokers were in college to party and be on vacation. I felt so ashamed when I arrived back at the house because it looked like I had just given up, but at the same time I was relieved. I felt like I had let my parents down by leaving school. I was and still am a fierce competitor at heart. I had to be, considering the magnitude of the physical and emotional suffering I had endured and overcome in my battles with lung disease. Yet my physical health and well-being was at stake, too, and I realized that I was not in the best physical shape and condition to live away from home in a dormitory to go to college and excel in my studies. Dormitory life was not the place for me to be so that I could get the proper rest I needed to attend classes, study and do homework, and succeed in getting a degree. A top priority was taking care of myself by getting my lungs stronger and healthier through proper diet and exercise.

Eventually my parents got me the counseling I needed, and I took aptitude tests to determine the right course of study and career. I had been leaning toward a career in law because I so thoroughly enjoyed the TV program *Perry Mason*, but the tests showed my aptitude for numbers and accounting. Mother and Daddy both were good in numbers and math. Later I would enroll in the School of Business Administration at Georgia State University in January 1969, majoring in Accounting and also minoring in Mathematics. I would live at home the entire time while I was attending Georgia State during the day. This university was famous for its night classes for those students who worked during the day.

I started to work out with my dad at the health club 2 or 3 times a week, and I also began to jog a few hundred yards slowly each day, weather permitting. What terrified me so was my constant fear and dread of suffering yet another collapsed lung. I was training and working out with totally no supervision whatsoever. Without any forethought I had to set boundaries and slowly but surely determine what my physical limitations actually were on a daily basis. I will never forget what Dirty Harry said in the final scene of the movie *Magnum Force* [1973] starring Clint Eastwood: **"A man's got to know his limitations"**. That was going to be the story of my life from now on.

During 1969 I joined the Atlanta Track Club and became a track and field official for high school track meets. Daddy and I began to jog together at the track of Headland High School. I did most of my running on the road near my house in East Point. My self-confidence and resolve increased as I began to get in a rhythm during my runs, and my conditioning and endurance soon followed suit. It took me 5 long years [March 1966 through January 1971] to recover from the trauma of lung disease. **On January 1, 1971 I ran 6 miles for the first time over a 3-mile cross country course in 43 minutes, 41 seconds. I had actually run with only 1 lung functioning,**

**my right lung. By no means a world record, but it was a miracle just the
same. I duplicated the feat on June 30, 1971.** In the summers of 1971 and
1973 the Atlanta Track Club sponsored an All-Comers Meet at Carling
Brewery. Daddy and I entered the father and son relay in both years, and we
finished in 2nd place each time. I missed the track and softball season in 1972
because of a nagging pulled groin muscle.

Later in life I was still actively running and staying in shape for playing
sports such as basketball and softball. I had played both basketball and
softball for Good Shepherd Lutheran Church in a church league in College
Park which seemed to make up for my lousy decision of quitting Little
League baseball after only playing 2 seasons. Sometimes I ran "splits" on
the track at Berkmar High School in Lilburn, Georgia. I ran 40 yard sprints
parallel to the football field, and I was regularly clocked under 4.5. My fastest
time was 4.25 in the 40. Just amazing considering I had survived 3 collapsed
lungs, and Dr. Mason Lowance, our family doctor, had told me I would
never run fast again! Dr. Lowance had run track and field at Washington
& Lee. Roy Hartsfield, mayor of Atlanta, was one of Dr. Lowance's famous
patients. My idols in track and field were Mel Pender, Houston McTear, Steve
Williams, John Carlos, Valeriy Borzov of the former Soviet Union, Jim Ryun,
Steve Prefontaine, John Akii-Bua of Uganda, and Kipchoge Keino of Kenya.
Borzov was the most efficient mechanical sprint champion that I have ever
seen and tried to emulate. My friends still do not believe I can run that fast.
But that is a fact because I know I have.

Today I suffer with chronic bronchiectasis and musculo skeletal pain.
I have also suffered with chronic lung infections ever since, including a
mycobacterial lung infection [*MAC*] diagnosed in July 2010. I think back
now on this long journey that I never gave it a thought that God was always
there with me each step of the way. I was just a young boy, but my mother
was always there praying for me constantly to get well. I am now reminded
of the passage in **Mark, Chapter 11, Verses 22 through 24 [New King
James Version]**, which proclaims the power of prayer:

> **"22 So Jesus answered and said to them, "Have faith in
> God. 23 For assuredly, I say to you, whoever says to this
> mountain, 'Be removed and be cast into the sea,' and
> does not doubt in his heart, but believes that those**

things he says will be done, he will have whatever he says. [24] Therefore I say to you, whatever things you ask when you pray, believe that you receive *them*, and you will have *them*."

This scripture is the basis for the expression **"having faith to move mountains"**. Mother was always my "port in the storm" and our family's beloved prayer warrior as well as residing "doctor".

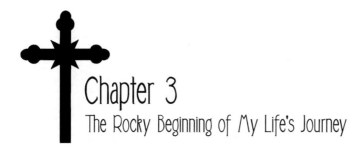

Chapter 3
The Rocky Beginning of My Life's Journey

September 5, 1973....

Mother cried the day I left to "forge my destiny" out in the real world down in Clearwater Beach, Florida. It was my first attempt to make it on my own since I had lived my entire life up until now in Atlanta. I had lived at home the entire time I went to Georgia State University. I had spent so much time on vacation in Florida that I became intoxicated by the Gulf of Mexico, the beaches, and the wildlife, especially the sea gulls, pelicans, different species of fish, the dolphins, and, of course, the bikini-clad sunbathers. My parents and I visited the Tampa Bay area prior to my decision to move, and I had discussed the employment opportunities in the area with Snelling & Snelling, an employment agency. During my visit, I did interview with Morgan Yacht Company about a cost accounting position. The job would have been fascinating since my job duties would involve the fabrication and assembly of the world famous yachts in their factory on Bryan Dairy Road in Clearwater. But at the time I was indecisive about whether or not to relocate for the first time in my life to a totally unfamiliar area where I did not know anyone.

I loaded what little belongings I had in my Ford Mustang and headed for Florida to start a new chapter in my life. I did not realize until much later that the Rolling Stones had composed their famous hit song *I Can't Get No (Satisfaction)* in 1965 at Clearwater Beach where I lived for a couple of weeks before I got a job and could rent an apartment on Missouri Avenue in Clearwater near Largo. On September 18, 1973, I was hired as the Staff Accountant in the Cash Receipts Department at Innisbrook Resort and Country Club in Tarpon Springs. Shirley Cox became my first supervisor. We were responsible for counting and recording the cash receipts at the front desk of the hotel and the country clubs as well as processing the proceeds generated from the sale of condominiums in buildings called lodges. In other words, we put money in the bank on a daily basis to keep the company running. In the hotel business there are no days off, even for holidays.

With what seemed to be a promising future with a job working for a well-managed company, I decided in January 1974 to purchase a condominium in Pinehurst Village in nearby Dunedin to establish my permanent residence and presumably live the rest of my life in the Tampa Bay area. It was the first home that I would own during my lifetime. I began my accounting "career" working extremely long hours. But I loved my job and the work I was doing despite the stress of daily deadlines in counting and processing the front desk receipts in time for pick up by the Brink's man for depositing in the bank. I maintained the monthly subsidiary ledgers containing the long-term debt of the company and the accrued interest due on these loans. I felt like I was contributing greatly to the success of the company, and I developed a sense of pride in paying the bills and covering the company payroll. This was a daily routine in our office, and at the end of the day we prepared the Daily Cash Report for the treasurer of the company, Richard Ferreira. This report summarized the total cash receipts as well as the cash disbursements by bank account, including payroll.

It was during the days at Georgia State and at this point in time of my life I developed my love of music. I used to play my 45's on Daddy's stereo system which I still have. He truly enjoyed listening to the Big Band music as well as Perry Como, Andy Williams, and Lawrence Welk. I could not get enough of *Abba,* the *Beatles,* the *Bee Gees, Chicago, Creedence Clearwater Revival, Doobie Brothers and Michael McDonald, Eagles, Elton John, Fleetwood Mac, The Rolling Stones* to name a few. Mother's favorite soft rock song, if there was one, was *Wildflower* (1973) by *Skylark.* Without music I believe I would have gone nuts because of the heavy workload and long hours and the disturbing health problems that loomed ahead in my immediate future.

Sometime during 1974 I began to have mysterious and increasing stomach discomfort and problems such as indigestion and upset stomach, especially while eating food. My primary physician diagnosed it as an ulcer and chronic gastritis which made my life absolutely miserable and troubling, considering the immense pressure I was constantly under at the office. My promotion shortly thereafter from Staff Accountant to Cash Receipts

Supervisor and Assistant to the Treasurer magnified the stress and tension I was facing at the company. Shirley Cox had decided to retire to spend more time with her husband, and I reluctantly replaced her. At that point I felt that I was already "married to my job". I started taking the medication Librax at each meal which was supposed to help me to digest food. My primary physician had prescribed Librax to reduce the symptoms of stomach and intestinal cramping by working to slow the natural movements of the gut and relaxing the muscles in the stomach and intestines. This medication also helps to reduce anxiety by acting on the brain and nerves to produce a calming effect. I had to stay away from soft drinks, a tall order for me. However, my stomach issues continued to persist.

To quote Jacob Riis, the 19th Century social reformer, **"[w]hen nothing seems to help, I go back and look at a stonecutter hammering away at his rock perhaps a hundred times without as much as a crack showing in it. Yet at the hundred and first blow it will split in two, and I know it was not that blow that did it—but all that had gone before."** So I continued to work out with weights as I had done back home in Atlanta. I was also running on the days that I did not work out with weights. This was going to turn out to be a fateful decision for my life and health because I realized daily exercise greatly relieves stress and tension. Over time, however, I had found that weightlifting and running on the same day were hard on my body. I had to let my body recover from the rigors of lifting weights. I would jump over the fence and run wind sprints on Dunedin High School's track. Somehow one day I was clocked in the 100 yard dash in a wind-aided 9.2. The world record for the 100 yard dash at that time was 9 flat.

What is so unbelievable is I was in superb physical condition during 1974 and 1975 as the direct result of working out and running on a regular basis. Sailing, fishing, and going to the beach always brought me peace and some sense of contentment and belonging. I regularly attended St. Paul's Lutheran Church in Clearwater. Daddy always said that the church is the best place to meet the right kind of people and enjoy a variety of activities such as Sunday School, Bible study, and sports. I bowled weekly in the company bowling league, and I even played basketball for St. Paul's Lutheran Church until I got so sick and dehydrated when I was battling a cold that I had to be put in Morton Plant Hospital in February 1975. I had been constantly vomiting and could not keep any food down, including water. I was so disoriented from the dehydration that my good friends Kaye and Theresa Neuman had to take me to the hospital. It is still so incredible to me that the hospital staff or my own family physician did not discover the swollen appendix that was festering inside my abdomen at that time. Trouble was the stomach pain and discomfort were emanating from the left side of my abdomen opposite to where the appendix is located. These symptoms had all the doctors totally baffled, including me. From this point on, the doctors have tended to have a difficult time in diagnosing and treating my future health problems. Mother, who had come down from Atlanta during this time, was there to take care of me as only she could do by fixing me home-cooked meals and taking me to the doctor or grocery store.

Before I left my boyhood home, Mother had given me a 3" by 5" card containing the following inspirational quotes:

I can do all things through Christ who strengthens me. [Philippians, Chapter 4, Verse 13.]

If I have faith and trust in the Lord, nothing is impossible unto me.

If God is with us, who can be against us? [Romans, Chapter 8, Verse 31.]

The Lord is my light and my salvation; whom shall I fear? The Lord is the strength of my life; in this will I be confident. [Psalm 27, Verse 1.]

We are always in God's hands.

God is our refuge and strength; a present help in time of trouble. [Psalm 46, Verse 1.]

Be still, and I know that I am God. [Psalm 46, Verse 10.]

At first I thought Mother herself had written these sayings just for me. I did not realize that they were scriptures from the Bible. I have since memorized them and recite them first thing in the morning and then at night before I go to bed. Then I pray for others who are suffering not only physically but also spiritually and emotionally or in need of a miracle.

After I left the hospital, I continued to have persistent stomach discomfort and gastritis. Medication or watching what I ate or drank did not help much. Even so, I resumed working out at the health club and running on the days I did not work out. My will to live was so relentless, and so was my growing faith in the Lord. I continued to work hard at the company and do my job faithfully, but I kept the seriousness of my illness a secret from everyone. I was thankful that I had such conscientious and hard-working employees like Kaye and Linda working under my supervision. I played for the championship softball team of St. Paul's Lutheran Church that went undefeated at 19-0 and won the regular season title in June 1975. I truly believe that sports and athletics are not only a great outlet for fun and fellowship with people from all walks of life but also a way to get in shape and stay healthy and strong. I still enjoyed sailing and swimming in the Gulf of Mexico. The sound of the surf is so intoxicating and soothing. This summer also was a time of sorrow when Punky, our fox terrier, passed away in July. She had lived 16 years with us and had been my faithful companion from my boyhood until I was a young adult at age 24.

In August 1975 God came to me as I was walking out the door to go to work one day. I can remember that encounter as if it was yesterday. Even though I was feeling so bad and so sick, God reassured me that I was going to be all right and just continue to live my life with faith in Him to give me strength and discernment each day. I truly believe my parents' prayers sustained me during these days of suffering and uncertainty. Earlier in the year I had resumed weekly massage therapy which I received from George LaFalgio at the health club in Clearwater. Over the years when I was attending Georgia State, I had received massage therapy during the time I was working out at the health club in Atlanta, and I would use the whirlpool to soothe sore muscles and for relaxation. George, who was a former boxer from New York City, helped me to stay relaxed and calm during the stressful times at the office. I enjoyed relaxing in the whirlpool, too, at the health club in Clearwater.

On September 15, 1975 I ran wind sprints after work in the subdivision where I lived. I still cannot believe I had been running that day. The next day I went to work as usual. I began to experience a stomach ache around 3:00PM which got worse and worse as the afternoon came to a close. I guess I ate some supper, and then I was determined to work out at the health club around 7:00PM. But I reluctantly decided not to go because my stomach pain was so much worse than before. By 11:00PM I realized I was in serious trouble, and I got dressed and drove myself to the emergency room 1 mile away at nearby Mease Hospital in Dunedin. I was in such agony that I was all bent over and could not possibly stand up straight as I walked into the hospital lobby. How I managed to drive to the hospital I do not know. All I can say is the Good Lord was my co-pilot. Fortunately for me there was no one else in the emergency room at that moment. The nurses took care of me immediately and placed me on a gurney, and X-rays were taken of my abdomen as soon as possible. The X-rays revealed a large cyst or possibly a tumor in my intestinal tract. The preliminary diagnosis was a possible gall stone obstructing my intestines or bowel. The attending physicians decided to move me by ambulance to Morton Plant Hospital. The paramedic in the ambulance apologized for having to stick a tube down my nose and throat because my stomach was so bloated it was about to implode. I gagged as the tube went down my nostril into my throat, and I vomited all the food in my stomach. I thought I was going to choke to death. But I knew by now that he had just saved my life. I am not sure whether I thanked him or not for his compassion because I was in shock and so scared. I could not talk at all because of the tube in my throat and esophagus. When I arrived at the hospital, I asked someone to call my friends Kaye, my co-worker, and Theresa, her sister, who also lived in Pinehurst Village to let them know what had happened. It was approximately 1:30AM when I was told my mother was on her way from Atlanta to be with me.

Dr. John Snelling, a general surgeon whose office was located in nearby Largo, was summoned to determine the nature and cause of the blockage causing the abdominal pain. Dr. Snelling looked at the X-rays and any lab tests performed by the hospital. Based upon his knowledge, experience, and intuition, Dr. Snelling suspected a ruptured appendix, but the large cyst or tumor mimicked a gall stone. Therefore, Dr. Snelling had a surgeon who specialized in the surgical procedures for removal of the gall bladder standing by just in case. What Dr. Snelling found during the operation was absolutely astounding. Mother told me that the surgeons had indeed found a ruptured appendix complicated by a large stone wedged inside my rectum and also the presence of gangrene all over my abdomen. Dr. Snelling said that this stone, which can sometimes form during appendicitis, had actually left an imprint on my rectum. According to him, it was one of the largest stones he had ever seen. I was so thankful to be alive and in the best of hands at the hospital.

But what is so chilling here was that I was not expected to live because the poison from the gangrene was in my blood stream and had possibly spread over my entire body. Mother later told me that I had a fever over 105 degrees caused by the gangrene in my abdomen, and I was being treated with heavy duty antibiotics. I have been told that my baldness could have been caused by the high fever which can destroy hair follicles in your scalp. I started losing my hair after the surgery. I remember the monitors and other devices in my hospital room and the IVs in my hands and drainage tubes in my abdomen. I still had the tube inserted down my nostril and my throat that made it so hard for me to swallow. I was not allowed to eat or drink anything, even water. I will never forget the kindness and compassion of a nurse who was taking care of me. I was burning up with fever, and I asked her if I could have a cup of water to drink. She said no, but I could have some ice. Those cups of ice during the night were the greatest gift I have ever received from anyone because it lifted my spirits and gave me hope. At that point I knew I was dying, but I now felt God's presence, and a peace came over me that I cannot explain. The scripture in **Joshua, Chapter 1, Verse 9** [**New King James Version**], comes to mind:

> "⁹ **Have I not commanded you? Be strong and be of good courage; do not be afraid, nor be dismayed, for the LORD your God *is* with you wherever you go.**"

This truly was the moment of truth for me.

After 3 long days following the surgery, I sat up in my hospital bed and looked out the window of my room for the first time since I arrived at the hospital. I felt like a million dollars because the poison in my body was gone. I have never felt that great in all my life which had been spared. My mother's prayers for healing and restoration had spared my life. I am still reminded of the passage in **Mark, Chapter 11, Verses 22 through 24** [**New King James Version**], which heralds the awesome power of prayer:

> "²² So Jesus answered and said to them, "Have faith in God. ²³ For assuredly, I say to you, whoever says to this mountain, 'Be removed and be cast into the sea,' and does not doubt in his heart, but believes that those things he says will be done, he will have whatever he says. ²⁴ Therefore I say to you, whatever things you ask when you pray, believe that you receive *them*, and you will have *them*."

As I think back on this experience, I remembered that part of the Apostles' Creed we recite during each church service: "**.....On the third day He [Jesus] rose again from the dead. He ascended into heaven and is seated at the right hand of God the Father Almighty....**" It was 3 days before I was able to get up out of bed and walk freely without IVs and tubes draped all over me. Kaye told me that Mother's hair had turned gray overnight because she knew I was so seriously ill and near death. Kaye and Theresa told me that they got "a kick out of being around my mother", and they remained friends throughout their lifetimes. Mother and I were always so close since I was an only child. I know how tough it had to be for my dad who had stayed behind in Atlanta to work. It took over a month for me to fully recover from the removal of my ruptured appendix and the stone in my abdomen and return to work. I was unable to work out at the health club or run.

Ironically in the past few months prior to the ruptured appendix, I had begun to glance at "help wanted ads" in the newspapers, checking out the job opportunities with better pay and, more importantly, shorter work hours. I loved my job and my co-workers at Innisbrook, but the stress and working long hours had taken its toll on my health, not only physically but also emotionally. I was "married to my job". All I was doing was eating, working, and sleeping. I had no social life. Life was passing me by. Earlier in the summer I had contacted Dan Alston who lives in Lilburn, Georgia outside Atlanta and had gone to school with me at Georgia State. We both had majored in accounting. Dan had an accounting job opening at Imperial Group Limited, the company where he was working at that time. This company was a hotel management firm, and I now had experience in the hotel industry which would be beneficial to perform the job duties and responsibilities of this accounting position.

While I was still in the hospital recovering from the surgery, I received a telephone call from Dan that this job was mine if I wanted it. I discussed the pros and cons of accepting this job offer with Mother and Daddy who were so concerned about my health and well-being. I realized that I would have to sell my condominium in Dunedin and then relocate to Atlanta which was going to be a great challenge to say the least. I literally had gotten another job while lying flat on my back in the hospital. I told Dan the story of what had happened to me and that I was still recuperating from the operation and its aftermath. He cautioned me to take my time to get well and regain my strength. During my recovery I worked at home on the accounting records of Innisbrook so that I would not be so far behind in my office work. Upon my return to the office, I tendered my resignation to the shock of everyone in the company.

The great tragedy about Florida living is the harsh reality that knocks you down when you look for employment in the Sunshine State. Salaries and wages are so much lower in Florida than the rest of the country despite the fact that the cost of living in Florida is so high. I always heard the comment that the sunshine and warm climate are part of your salary. But the sun and warm temperatures won't pay the rent or put food on the table. The huge supply of labor in the state allows employers to hire anyone off the streets at whatever wage they want to pay. It seems like employers do not mind paying you a low wage because there are so many people looking for employment that you are indeed expendable and replaceable. In fact, I was told on a number of occasions that I was "overqualified" for the position I was applying for. Plentiful jobs abound for those in the construction industry and the health care, legal, and real estate professions. A classic example of the plight of a Florida resident who is not retired and not living on Social Security and pensions or wealth and riches is the personnel system of the Florida Department of Revenue which was created in 1968. Do the math. That's almost 50 years ago. As an employee in Florida state government, you are at the mercy of the state legislature who determines the pay scales or grades as well as pay raises. I recently had a conversation with a gentleman whom I was a caregiver for, and he made the comment that you better take a large sum of money with you if you want to live in Florida because you will never make any down there. Food for thought for those of you who are thinking about moving to the Sunshine State.

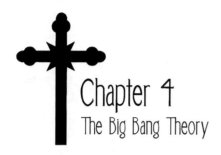

Chapter 4
The Big Bang Theory

November 1975....

After my return to Atlanta from living 2 years in the Tampa Bay area, I started the new accounting job with my friend Dan Alston at Imperial Group Limited, a hotel management firm near Stone Mountain. After 4 months working with Dan, I could see "the writing on the wall" that the company appeared to be in serious financial trouble. Again I started to scour the "help wanted ads" and update my resume. At that time my dad was working as the Credit Manager of Fulton Supply Company in downtown Atlanta, and he got a telephone call from his close friend John Herron that J. M. Tull Metals Company, a metals service center, was looking for a General Accountant. I interviewed with Warren Pass who was the controller of J. M. Tull, and I was eventually selected for the accounting position. On March 15, 1976, I began my career at the company. Working under Mr. Pass in the Finance Department, I was responsible as the company's sales tax specialist. I assisted in the preparation of the weekly and monthly payrolls when needed as a backup for the Payroll Administrator and financial statements. I reconciled all major bank accounts and performed the internal audit function in connection with Accounts Payable. The company moved from Marietta Street across from the famous Omni International Hotel in downtown Atlanta to Norcross shortly after I started to work there. I eventually moved from my parents' house in East Point into a one bedroom apartment in Norcross. I still had my fiery red Ford Mustang in the parking lot. I quickly found out that "apartment living" was not for me. The neighbor next door playing his stereo at 3:00AM in the morning, someone stealing the entire taillight housing from my car out in the parking lot, the size of the apartment that was so small you had to go outside to change your mind.

Spring of 1977....

I heard that J. M. Tull had a softball team that played at Best Friend Park in Norcross, and I decided to play softball in March 1977 after skipping the season following the 1975 championship season in Florida. At that time I met Johnie Tumlin who worked in the Atlanta warehouse, and we became teammates as well as friends. During the season our manager left the team, and I felt compelled for whatever reason to take over the management of the team. I consider this decision to be the turning point of my life. As the manager I had to take charge and become more assertive and self-confident in putting the team together and making decisions. Clarence Irwin was the personnel manager whom I had a long conversation with about the future and benefits of having a softball team for the employees. With the assistance of Mr. Irwin we began to rebuild the softball program. I focused on building a strong infield with great pitching and the catcher and strong centerfielder up the middle. I moved to play first base, and the rest is history. Johnie got us permission to practice at Ocee Elementary School near Alpharetta. From that point on, the team record was 7-6, and we actually sponsored softball tournaments in the summers of 1977 and 1978. We were able to assemble strong competitive teams with great players, and our team finished in 2nd place in our Industrial League in 1979 and 1981. With the support of the company we were able to build a softball field during 1980 for all employees to enjoy.

After living in the small apartment for a year in Norcross, I moved into a brick duplex apartment in Lawrenceville for the next 6 years. I was 27 years old at the time, and life was good. I had a **"world at my feet" mentality**. I was dating up a storm and playing sports and working out with weights. I was in superb physical condition, considering my past history of lung and respiratory problems. I was running every other day and feeling great about my life and what it had to offer. I was beginning to plan to "settle down", get married, and start a family of my own. I had 2 special ladies in my life during 1980 and 1981, and the possibility of married life and raising a family looked promising indeed. I still think about the special lady named Bonnie and whether or not God had placed her in my life for a purpose. I was just getting to know Bonnie.

Carol Hunt will always be the first love of my life even though we were both young children when we were growing up together in East Point. **Like in the movies, Carol was literally "the girl next door".** Why Carol did not pursue a career in modeling I do not know because she was so beautiful. I was always hindered by my lack of self-confidence and self-esteem in my earlier days in school. I noticed that girls were only interested in me because I could help them with their homework. For example, I remember Lorraine, a beautiful brunette in elementary school, who asked me to help her with a project. I really was attracted to this girl. However, all she was interested in was getting her homework done. I also liked Katie in elementary school because I thought she reminded me so much of Mother, but this girl did not even give me the time of day. I began to realize that most girls were only interested in my so-called intellect and knowledge, not as a boy to get to know and be a friend with. I became so depressed about potential relationships with girls. What did I have to offer them? To this day I am still baffled by what women want. I tended to put women on a pedestal because my mother was such a saint in my eyes, and I thought that women had to be similar to her. I had such a crush on Maureen McCormick, the actress, who played Marcia Brady on *The Brady Bunch*. I remember my parents and I were at the airport one night. We were walking to the gate when I spotted Maureen McCormick and the rest of *The Brady Bunch* sneaking through the airport trying not to be noticed. She is still such a beautiful lady today.

I can honestly say that I am a "late bloomer" when it comes to the dating scene and learning how to build relationships. What was so devastating about my school years was the grueling recovery from 3 collapsed lungs that I suffered in March 1966 and March 1967. I did not even attend the junior and senior proms in high school because of my poor health. Physical adversity had obviously been such a major factor in the total disruption of my social life as a teenager. It is difficult to be yourself when you do not feel well and are suffering emotionally as well as physically. During my college days I had little or no time for dating. Majoring in accounting and minoring in mathematics and history, I had to study long, long hours just to get my BBA degree at Georgia State University. Dennis, who attended Georgia Tech, was kind enough to set me up with a few dates which did not materialize into anything special for me or the lady. I was so naïve and unassertive when it came down to women and what they are looking for in a relationship. Of course, I had never been on my own to start learning about what life is really all about and to be responsible for myself until after my graduation from Georgia State University in June 1973. My job at Innisbrook Resort as the Assistant to the Treasurer and Cash Receipts Supervisor gave me no time to even think about romance. The suffering and discomfort I endured with the upset stomach caused by a diseased appendix during 1974 and most of 1975 made it so difficult for me to work hard and stay employed much less recreate or socialize. I was under extremely intense pressure working with the Treasurer to run the company. But I do remember Linda, a beautiful blue-eyed blonde who worked with me.

I had decided to put a personal ad in the *Atlanta Singles Magazine* containing a brief profile of myself. I received several responses to my ad from ladies who briefly told me about themselves and invited me to contact them if I was interested in meeting and getting to know them. I will never forget the letter I received from a young lady that I will call Lee who responded to my personal ad. When I first met her, it was love at first sight for me. **Lee was 22 and only 5' 2" inches tall, but she had beautiful, soft jet black hair and the beauty of Jaclyn Smith to boot.** I guess I had a crush on Jaclyn Smith, too. My Aunt Emily told me that when I met the right lady, it would "feel like a load of bricks had fallen on me". She was right as she always was.

On our next date Lee was so delighted and excited that we were going to the roller skating rink. She really enjoyed skating, but I have always had 2 left feet when it comes to skating or dancing for that matter. I really was in love with Lee, and I kissed her for the first time at the skating rink. I felt like I was on Cloud 10. When I kissed her again, she had to stand up on the door step because I am a foot taller than she is. The tragedy of it all was she did not feel the same way I did about her, but I was too blind to see it. Lee told me that I was "getting too serious", but I felt that she was just toying with my emotions. I was truly smitten by this girl. She claimed that she was not going to get married any time soon. A few months later, Lee called me at the office and informed me *over the telephone* that she was getting married to a guy named Richard. I was so heartbroken. **The greatest compliment I ever received from her is that I am level-headed.**

It may be hard to believe but not one time did I ever sleep with anyone or ever desire to do so. I want to save that moment of joy for my wedding night. **What I have found quite often is women find me too good to be true.** I have been told that quite a few times, too many times actually. I am no saint and never claimed to be. I do not walk on water. But several lessons I have learned from all these experiences. My personality has blossomed so much in my later years as I have become a good conversationalist, more relaxed and self-confident, and feel more comfortable with my sense of humor and love of laughter. I now try to focus on activities that the lady wants to do and enjoy. I deeply regret that I did not go out with Bonnie anymore than I did. She stays in my mind because she accepted me for who I am, a quality Christian man. No pretense whatsoever.

October 8, 1981....

Just another unremarkable day in what would begin a remarkable story of triumph over unconscionable pain and suffering, bitterness, anger, fear, and a test of my faith and belief in God's grace and mercy. It was about 7:30 in the morning, and for some inexplicable reason I was having difficulty getting dressed and putting the cap back on the tooth paste. After combing what little hair I had on my head, I was on my way out the door to go to work at J. M. Tull Metals Company 8 miles away on Buford Highway.

My fabled bright red 1966 Ford Mustang and beautiful turquoise blue 1977 Ford Mustang awaited me in the driveway. I called the carport of my duplex apartment my "corral" for my "ponies". I had saved my money since childhood to buy my first Mustang which was my pride and joy. I did odd jobs, sold cokes to carpenters and bricklayers building new houses in our neighborhood, and collected empty coke bottles discarded along the side of the road to redeem the deposits. Topp Cola bottles were highly prized for taking to nearby grocery stores to cash them in. I paid only $1,900 for the car that I bought from a nurse through a dealer. **The nurse had decided to trade in the Ford Mustang for a Corvair.** Imagine that! The original color of the car was white, but I decided to have it repainted red to match the black leather bucket seats. I called this Mustang the *Red Baron*, and I named the other Mustang the *Blue Max* since I am part German.

I made the fateful decision to drive my "old friend" to the office that day. In her day the 1966 Mustang was well-built and already a classic automobile. I had owned the car since late 1968 during my freshman year in college. As I drove closer and closer to the office, I was going around a curve in the road. I was only 2 miles from the office when I felt God's presence that warned me of the danger approaching down the road. A month earlier I had had a premonition about the tragic auto accident that was going to violently interrupt my life and almost end it. Halfway around the curve God told me to slow down. A white 1963 Rambler station wagon swerved over the center line of the road and plowed into my car. I tried desperately to steer away from the oncoming car, but to no avail. For years later I had nightmares about the accident, and from that point I was terrified whenever a vehicle would veer ever so slightly or swerve to the median of a road or highway. The trauma of the accident still haunts me to this day. I guess it always will.

Most of my friends and fellow employees thought that it was a "fender bender". **The head-on collision with the drunk driver was no "fender bender".** The car crash destroyed my Ford Mustang and nearly ended my life. I will never forget the kindness of drivers who were behind me at the time of the accident and my fellow employees, Warren Pass, the controller, and Cris Tarquinio who came to my aid on the roadside near Buford Highway. It was so disgusting that the drunk driver was more concerned about discarding the Budweiser he had stashed in his coolers in the station wagon that had slammed into my car than me and my welfare. I remember his appearance to be that of a homeless, disheveled man who was filthy from head to toe. I do not remember if the drunk driver ever apologized or showed any concern or remorse about my well-being and injuries. I was embittered for a long time that this man had ruined my life. It is tragic it took so many years to change the attitudes of the public, news media, lawmakers, and law enforcement that drunk driving is indeed a crime. However, I began to pray that this drunk driver would never be allowed to hurt anyone else. With these prayers to God eventually came forgiveness and a sense of peace so that I could move on with my own life. I have learned that you have to let go of anger and bitterness by forgiving the person who has wronged you and leave it up to God to take care of the rest. God is the ultimate judge and no respecter of persons.

It has haunted me relentlessly that I was not wearing a seat belt. Remember, at that time Georgia state law did not require drivers to wear seat belts, and it was 8 o'clock in the morning for heaven's sake. Even though I was in superb physical condition at the time of the accident, I suffered a severe concussion and neck injuries when I tried to exit the windshield upon impact. My lower back, left hip, and left knee were also injured when my body was slammed into the dashboard. Two of my front teeth were also badly chipped. **When the Aetna insurance agent representing the drunk driver met with me, he had the audacity to tell me....**"**Mr. Hime, you were just in the wrong place at the wrong time.**" I was so upset by what I had said to me, and I let him know how much I was suffering at the time. But as I look back at the terrible injuries caused by the accident, I thank the Lord that I did not end up like Christopher Reeve who was paralyzed from the neck down after falling off a horse. Yet as time went on I became more and more frustrated and exasperated with my circumstances and suffered from bouts of depression and despair.

Unfortunately the auto accident fell under the infamous "no fault" insurance coverage which was in force in Georgia during 1981. At the time of the accident, my insurance carrier was Wausau Underwriters' Insurance Company. By definition **no-fault insurance** is a type of car insurance in which an insurance provider covers damages incurred to its customer in an accident, regardless of who is at fault. According to Allstate Insurance Company, this type of insurance coverage essentially eliminates the need for a driver to go after another party's insurance company in order to be reimbursed for damages that the other person caused. No-fault car insurance is currently in place in 12 states and the Commonwealth of Puerto Rico. What exactly does this type of insurance cover?

Bodily injury. Traditional car insurance policies let you take out liability coverage to pay for bodily injury claims from anyone injured in an accident in which you have been deemed at fault. With no-fault car insurance, the bodily injury coverage provided by your policy extends to you. One of the benefits of having no-fault coverage is that medical claims are paid quickly and you don't have to wait for a lawsuit before you are reimbursed for money you would otherwise have to pay out of pocket for your medical expenses.

Associated medical bills and other losses. The Personal Injury Protection element of no-fault car insurance ensures not only that your hospital bills are paid, but that you're also covered for any associated losses. For example, if you are injured and unable to return to work for some time, your no-fault coverage may help foot the bill for lost wages. This is not always a guarantee, and availability varies by state.

What Does No-Fault Insurance Not Cover? The term "no-fault" usually pertains only to coverage relating to personal injury and does not include coverage for property damage. In states that require consumers to have a no-fault car insurance policy, as in states without no-fault insurance, the liability coverage in your auto insurance policy covers you for damages to another person's car, and you can purchase collision coverage for your own vehicle.

I deliberated for quite awhile as to what to do about the impact of the insurance coverage upon my physical well-being and the cost of future medical treatment and care for my injuries. **Remember: Under No-fault insurance, the bodily injury coverage provided by your insurance policy extends to you. One of the benefits of having no-fault coverage is that medical claims are paid quickly, and you do not have to wait for a lawsuit before you are reimbursed for money you would otherwise have to pay out of pocket for your medical expenses**. Based upon this interpretation of the insurance policy and its coverage provisions, I decided not to proceed with legal action against the drunk driver or his brother-in-law whose automobile he was driving.

Compounding my decision was the devastating and crippling effects of the severe concussion that adversely affected my judgment for weeks on end. For a long time I could not add 2 and 2. I have read magazine articles about the nature and diagnosis of concussions, including those published in *Sports Illustrated* about football players. From what I understand, there is no such thing as a slight or mild concussion. It is like being pregnant. Either you are or you are not. As I have said before, I suffered my first concussion in 1960 at the age of 10 during a "touch" football game during recess at elementary school. Later in my youth, I crashed my head into the bottom of the backboard when I was playing basketball, and I saw "stars" and had a large bump or crease on my head resulting in a nasty headache afterwards.

My worst concussion was my last that occurred in the head-on collision with the drunk driver. When I was propelled into the windshield upon impact, the blow to my head caused a permanent lump on the left side of my head. I have no memory of what happened next after the crash. Later on after the accident I found a piece of my scalp on the seal of the windshield, confirming what my head had actually hit. Again I was so dazed and unsteady on my feet that I had to be helped to walk away from the scene of the accident. Someone alerted me to turn off the engine of my car which I did not even realize was still running because I was so in a daze and shock.

I had such a terrible headache and was not allowed to sleep more than 1 hour at a time the night of the accident. What still boggles my mind is that I was not admitted into the hospital that dreadful day but was released despite the fact that I had suffered a severe concussion and an injury to my left knee in the automobile accident. My left knee had apparently slammed into the dashboard upon impact. I had a large knot on my knee which had hit one of the knobs on the dashboard so hard it was bent upward. My left knee has bothered me ever since. At times I have suffered loss of memory and concentration, blackouts, headaches, acute sinusitis, and pain in my head around the area where I struck the windshield. I made the crucial decision to concentrate on using my insurance coverage to pay for medical expenses related to the automobile accident and regain my health through any means necessary. What I never perceived or could ever imagine was the long, painful, agonizing journey that I was about to embark upon not only to diagnose and treat my injuries but also to find myself and go on with the rest of my life.

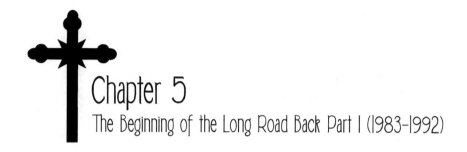

Chapter 5
The Beginning of the Long Road Back Part I (1983–1992)

I had no idea of the magnitude and severity of the injuries I had suffered in the accident. I am thankful to this day that I was in superb physical condition at the time of the accident. Otherwise, I would have had a broken neck or worse and been killed instantly. When my head apparently hit the seam of the windshield, I suffered not only a severe concussion but also TMJ after my face had slammed into the steering wheel, damaging my jaw and front teeth in the process. It is heartbreaking to me now that it took 11 years to diagnose TMJ or TMD in November 1992 by Dr. John Hughes, a dentist.

The winter of 1982 was extremely cold and frigid. The Atlanta area experienced bitter cold temperatures and snow and sleet storms. One of the lowest temperatures ever recorded here was 5 degrees below zero on January 11, 1982. The wind chill was clocked at 37 degrees below zero. The next day the Atlanta area was hit by a major snowstorm which was nicknamed Snow Jam 1982. With bitter, arctic cold air in place, a frigid ground, and moisture moving in, the stage was set for something epic. Heavy snow started falling just before rush hour on Tuesday, January 12, 1982. Every single flake that fell "stuck". Many commuters like me who started home never made it with their vehicles. Some were forced to stay the night at their place of work. I had to leave my 1977 Ford Mustang parked in a ditch on the side of the road and walk to my parents' house over a mile away with a severe cold and sore throat. The temperature was a frigid 21 degrees, but I had no choice but to abandon my car at the bottom of a steep hill before I could cross the railroad tracks.

Medical science and technology was just beginning to evolve in 1981 into what it is today. Initially, for the first few weeks, Wausau Underwriters Insurance Company, my insurance carrier at the time of the accident, authorized and paid for extensive physical therapy for my back pain and discomfort which helped me for a short period of time. But I began to suffer more and more as the days and weeks wore on. What was so devastating was I was no longer able to run well and work out at the health club like I did before the accident so that I could continue to take care of myself as usual. Without my parents I would have not survived the physical adversity, pain, and suffering I unknowingly was going to face and endure for many, many years to come. I had to relearn how to work out with weights which had been such an asset in the past to take care of myself. Now I was dealing with physical limitations in lifting weights. Even picking up a piece of paper off the floor could "throw my back out". Up until the accident I had been working out regularly at the health club. I could leg press 500 pounds, lift 300 pounds on the thigh extension machine, squat 250 pounds, and lift 600 pounds on the toe raise machine. I could easily do over 12 "pull downs" with 120 pounds of weight. Even considering my past health history of lung and abdominal surgeries, I was a powerful athlete in superb physical condition. Believe or not, I could consistently run the 40 yard dash under 4.5 seconds. At Berkmar High School in Lilburn, I was clocked in the 40 at 4.25 seconds. But by the fall of 1981 this was all going to change with the blink of an eye. As I look back, the biggest mistake I made was playing the 1982 softball season with J. M. Tull with a painful back and left hip injury. I had no business playing softball which I know now further damaged my back and could have caused catastrophic life-changing consequences bordering on potential paralysis and disability.

The frigid weather of 1982 and the following winter of 1983 fueled my desire to relocate to the warmer climate of the Tampa Bay area which I had enjoyed during the 1970's. Years before in the 1960's, my parents had decided to purchase lots from General Development Corporation [GDC] located in Port Charlotte and Port St. Lucie, Florida after checking out glossy brochures given by GDC and sales promotions by such celebrities as Arthur Godfrey. In *Wikipedia, the Free Encyclopedia [January 26, 2017]*, Elliot, Robert, and Frank Mackle Jr. founded GDC in Miami, Florida during 1954, and the company grew to become the largest developer of real estate in the state. During the next 2 decades, GDC developed several new properties, and the company pursued global advertising of its affordable home sites in the Sunshine State. Home and lot sales soared after GDC decided to give customers a "money back guarantee" on their purchases and promote a program whereby an undeveloped lot owner could exchange his property for developed real estate. GDC could now build new homes on a more timely and controlled basis. We swapped our undeveloped lots for a house that already been built by GDC as a "spec" home in North Port Charlotte, Florida. It was the first time in my life that I had had the opportunity to purchase a house but only with the help from my parents as co-owners.

Shortly before I moved to the Sarasota area, I had a **CT scan** performed on my lower back on June 23, 1983 at Northside Hospital in Atlanta which discovered only a bulging disc. **The test results of the scan read as follows: "There is posterior bulging of the disc interspace at the L4-5 level producing extrinsic compression of the ventral aspect of the fecal sac best appreciated on scan slice 16. There is minimal bulging of the disc interspace at the L5-S1 level without appreciable compression of the ventral aspect of the thecal sac at this latter level. There are no other findings to indicate the presence of a herniated nucleus pulposus..... CONCLUSION: Posterior bulging of the annulus fibrosis at the L4-5 level producing extrinsic compression of the ventral aspect of the thecal sac at this level."** In July 1983 I quit my accounting job at J. M. Tull, and I moved to North Port Charlotte outside Sarasota, Florida, thinking that my chronic pain and backache would benefit from the warmer climate and cleaner air. I had suffered so much during the frigid winters of 1982 and 1983 in the Atlanta area. In actuality I had basically given up on life itself. Florida had always been my haven and refuge in my youth, a source of happy times and fond memories.

It took a long time for me to come to the realization that I must **focus upon the activities that I can do without any discomfort, not the activities I cannot do.** I began to read the Bible more and more, and I found great solace, encouragement, and inspiration in reading Psalms and also **Verses 4-13 in Chapter 4 of Philippians [New King James Version]** which read as follows:

> **[4] Rejoice in the Lord always. Again I will say, rejoice! [5] Let your gentleness be known to all men. The Lord *is* at hand. [6] Be anxious for nothing, but in everything by prayer and supplication, with thanksgiving, let your requests be made known to God; [7] and the peace of**

God, which surpasses all understanding, will guard your hearts and minds through Christ Jesus. [8] Finally, brethren, whatever things are true, whatever things *are* noble, whatever things *are* just, whatever things *are* pure, whatever things *are* lovely, whatever things *are* of good report, if *there is* any virtue and if *there is* anything praiseworthy—meditate on these things. [9] The things which you learned and received and heard and saw in me, these do, and the God of peace will be with you. [10] But I rejoiced in the Lord greatly that now at last your care for me has flourished again; though you surely did care, but you lacked opportunity. [11] Not that I speak in regard to need, <u>for I have learned in whatever state I am, to be content:</u> [12] <u>I know how to be abased, and I know how to abound. Everywhere and in all things I have learned both to be full and to be hungry, both to abound and to suffer need.</u> [13] <u>I can do all things through Christ who strengthens me.</u>"

I tried to continue to work out with weights and jog, but both were a painful process because it was so difficult to find a combination of exercises and weights that did not aggravate my back. With the lower back and hip injuries, jogging jarred my back and drastically reduced my stride. I still remember what Dirty Harry said in the movie *Magnum Force* [1973]: **"A man's got to know his limitations"**. What an understatement. Colon problems also made my life absolutely miserable after the auto accident due to my weak back or so I thought. Several doctors' appointments later uncovered that I was lactose intolerant, and I had to stop drinking milk and eating ice cream for the first time in my life. Dairy products were basically off limits.

I started making regular trips to the chiropractor in Port Charlotte as I had previously done under the chiropractic care of Dr. John Glaccum in Lilburn, Georgia. Wausau Underwriters Insurance Company was still continuing to pay for the health care. I had never had a back injury as serious, debilitating, and nagging as this injury was and has been. Believe or not, 4 out of 5 people will experience back problems during their lifetimes. Lifting anything off the floor, toting groceries, mowing the lawn, bending over the sink to wash my hands, sitting for any length of time, making up the bed, even sneezing or coughing became an adventure. One time I noted during a doctor visit that I had hurt my back when I had a nightmare which caused me to jump out of bed. I asked the chiropractors about taking care of my back, and their advice was **not to reinjure it**. I suffered with an injury to the L5 and S1 vertebrae in my lower back which is a common injury for most people when they hurt their backs and spine.

Complicating matters was my inability and frustration in trying to find another job despite career counseling and extensive research into the job opportunities and the types of businesses prevalent in the area before we made the decision to relocate. I even thought about starting my own business mowing lawns and landscaping as well as sharpening tools. But I was unsure whether or not my health would hold up. At that time I had **no health insurance coverage** so I was taking great risk with my shaky health situation. I must have filled out a million job applications, but the all too common response from potential employers was I was overqualified for the positions advertised. In November 1983 I filled out an application for a tax auditor position with the Florida Department of Revenue in Sarasota, and Jesse Poston, the audit group supervisor, said he would contact me when there was an opening. I was searching for an employer who offered great fringe benefits such as group health insurance and a pension. I had planted a seed for a future that would unfold in less than a year.

In the meanwhile life goes on, and I finally got an accounting job with Arrow Aluminum, Inc. in December 1983 after 6 months of unemployment. I literally became the office manager, answering the telephone to talk with customers and suppliers; helping unload delivery trucks; paying the bills; preparing the weekly payroll, and communicating with the work crews and sales personnel out in the field. My top salary at Arrow Aluminum was only $15,000 a year with no fringe benefits compared with the annual salary of roughly $20,000 at J. M. Tull. My fringe benefit at Arrow Aluminum was just my paycheck I was told. I was eventually laid off by Arrow Aluminum in August 1984 after just 9 months of employment.

After my layoff, my dad and I were out in the sailboat in the Gulf of Mexico when we were ambushed by what locals call a "no name" storm. The winds were so fierce that the rain was coming down horizontally in my face, and our sailboat was being pushed backwards with the tidal surge. I was so scared when this vicious storm actually knocked out our boat motor. The storms of life hit us when we are so vulnerable and least expect them. But God is still in control, and we survived what could have been called a "small hurricane". The seas on which we are sailing once seemed so calm but are now chaotic and uncontrollable. Are we at the mercy of the wind and the water? As despair sets in, is all hope lost? I had just lost my job, and I thought seriously about returning to Atlanta because job opportunities were so scarce in the local area where we were living. I had serious health issues with my lower back and left hip. In the midst of a desperate situation, God never forsakes and leaves us to the mercy of the elements, but instead we are gathered in the embrace of a loving God. He is with you, especially when the wind changes and life gets hard. In **Second Corinthians, Chapter 12, Verses 9-10 [New King James Version]**, God offers us His free and unmerited favor:

> "⁹ **And He said to me, "My grace is sufficient for you, for My strength is made perfect in weakness." Therefore most gladly I will rather boast in my infirmities, that the power of Christ may rest upon me. ¹⁰ Therefore I take pleasure in infirmities, in reproaches, in needs, in persecutions, in distresses, for Christ's sake. For when I am weak, then I am strong."**

In all circumstances, when we lean on God for strength and help, we are truly strong. Fortunately after the storm we were towed back to the dock by another boat who saw us stranded. But I did not realize that this moment was going to be the turning point of my life. While my dad and I were out in the sailboat, I received the fateful telephone call from Jesse Poston who informed my mother that a tax auditor position was available at the Sarasota office of the Florida Department of Revenue. He told me to come in for an interview, and the rest is history.

With the refusal of Wausau Underwriters Insurance Company to provide further coverage of my medical treatments for my lower back and hip injuries during 1985, I began to consider other alternatives. My health insurance coverage was now under the State of Florida group policy with Blue Cross/Blue Shield, and I now felt I had a new lease on life. I visited Shands Memorial Hospital in Gainesville, Florida which is world renowned for its orthopedic staff and health care. I was so devastated when the neurosurgeons and doctors there scoffed at me and recommended "pain management" for my future health care. How dare you come here for medical treatment and advice when you at least can still walk and go to work every day! What's your problem? My main complaint was the quality of life and the pain that I was living with and the prognosis for the healing of my lower back and left hip. I had to turn this disappointment into an appointment.

On August 4, 1986 I made the critical decision to have a MRI performed on my lower back at the NMR Scanning Center in St. Petersburg, Florida to determine not only the nature and severity of the back and hip injury but also what potential options could be considered for medical and health care treatment. According to *WebMd.com* [*March 20, 2017*], magnetic resonance imaging (MRI) is a computerized test that uses a strong magnet in conjunction with radio waves and with or without contrast material to detect and diagnose health problems caused by cancer, tumors, injuries such as torn ligaments or broken bones, bleeding, and infection. Magnetic resonance imaging produces digital images that can be archived on a computer and can enhance and expand the information contained in the images taken by an X-ray, ultrasound, or CT scan. Areas of the body that can be imaged by MRIs include the head and brain, heart and lungs, blood vessels, bones and joints (including the temporomandibular joint), spine and lower back (bulging discs), and abdomen. It may be possible to have an MRI with an open machine that does not enclose your entire body.

John Rhodes, my good friend at Christ the King Lutheran Church, underwent surgery and subsequent chemotherapy treatments for colon and bladder cancer. For 10 years John had MRIs to confirm and ensure that he stayed in remission from cancer. The test results of my MRI using a standard MRI machine reaffirmed that I was not suffering with a herniated disc or damaged nerves in my lower back. It was so gratifying and a relief to know that I only had a bulging disc. Unfortunately I had to stop jogging on January 29, 1988 after 20 years of running at least 3 days a week to alleviate my respiratory problems and for my overall health and well-being. I had also discovered a long time ago while working at Innisbrook that running and exercising were great stress "busters" and a way of releasing nervous energy. However, running was jarring my lower back and hips so badly I had to discontinue it. I was beginning to explore all the options that I had at my disposal at that point in time.

One day my dad saw a newspaper article in the *Sarasota Herald-Tribune* about a man named David Shue who was well-known for 29 years throughout the Sarasota area as a master of **neuromuscular massage therapy.** I have learned that Shue passed away on July 16, 2010 at the age of 62. Believe it or not, **Shue had been completely blind since he was 12 years old. He had lost his eye sight when a "cherry bomb" firecracker exploded in his face.** I still remember the Australian shepherd, his faithful guide dog, who was always by his side. During my college days, I had had 2 other blind men work on me, but they were not neuromuscular massage therapists like he was. Shue had a gift as a motivational speaker because he loved to help and encourage others. I started to see him in March 1988, and his neuromuscular massage therapy in combination with workouts with Nautilus exercise equipment had given me enormous relief from the back pain and discomfort that I had experienced for so many years. But not a complete and lasting cure and solution to the elimination of my back pain.

Shue concentrated on the treatment of the piriformis which is a flat, band-like muscle located in the buttocks near the top of the hip joint. This muscle plays such a pivotal role in enabling us to walk, shift our weight from one foot to another, and maintain balance by stabilizing the hips and maneuvering the thighs away from the body. In other words. the piriformis muscle governs almost every motion of the hips and legs. The Piriformis Syndrome is a rare neuromuscular disorder caused by the compression of the piriformis upon the sciatic nerve which runs along or passing through the piriformis. A spasm within the piriformis can result in sciatic nerve pressure.

Under *Spine-health.com [March 20, 2017]*, **neuromuscular massage therapy** is highly regarded for its effectiveness for the treatment of lower back pain, especially soft tissue injuries like I suffered in the automobile accident. Patients with sore or injured muscles that are in spasm react to massaging these areas because of the pain and sensitivity in the tissues. Soreness in muscles is caused by the buildup of lactic acid which results from the lack of oxygen. The muscle spasm interferes with the flow of blood in the tissue and, therefore, deprives the muscle from getting enough oxygen. Neuromuscular massage therapy involves the application of the therapist's hands, knuckles, and even elbows, using different amounts of pressure upon the muscle spasm. Massage should relieve the muscle spasm unless inflammation is present. The release of lactic acid that results from massage therapy should, in turn, allow improved blood flow and oxygen in the affected muscle tissues. Neuromuscular massage therapists always instruct their patients to drink plenty of water to "flush out" the lactic acid. Please check out *Spine-health.com* for more information.

Neuromuscular massage therapy will produce the best results when combined with medical treatments such as physical therapy, chiropractic, or physician care. Numerous massage therapists will work in tandem with a multidimensional health care team in overall patient evaluation and treatment. **I owe a debt of gratitude that I can never repay to neuromuscular massage therapists such as David Shue, Carol Trescott in Tallahassee, and Paula Parcheta, Brenda Sheffield, and Jill Knueppel in the Atlanta area who have been so instrumental in turning my life around with neuromuscular massage therapy. I am living proof that neuromuscular massage therapy works.**

The key to my continuing comeback from the injuries suffered in the automobile accident was the eventual combination of neuromuscular massage therapy with prolotherapy for the medical treatment of the injured sacroiliac or sacral ligaments. I originally hurt my coccyx or tailbone in 1971 when I was lifting heavy weights one night on the leg press machine as well as later on when I was lifting a television set out of my car. According to *Spine-health.com [March 20, 2017]*, it was commonly believed that the coccyx consists of 3 to 5 separate or fused vertebrae at the end of the spinal column. The coccyx, however, does exhibit limited movement between the bones that is controlled by joints and ligaments since it is not one complete bone and is also connected to the sacrum with ligaments. These ligaments allow limited movement between the coccyx and the sacrum. When I was exercising with the leg press at the time of injuring my tailbone, I felt a twinge of pain right at the tailbone area. What I now believe is the pain in the coccyx was caused by the excessive pressure I had placed upon the area that forces the bones to move beyond their normal but limited range of motion. An injury to the coccyx can cause pain and result in inflammation. Again, please check out *Spine-health.com* for more information, including an article "The Anatomy of the Coccyx" written by Dr. Richard A. Staehler.

After numerous discussions with health care professionals and my own extensive research covering the medical treatment available for lower back injuries, I discovered Dr. Ben E. Benjamin who has dedicated his life to helping people cope with and overcome the pain and stress caused by injury to the body. His therapeutic techniques help reduce and eliminate pain produced by adhesive scar tissue formed from **soft tissue injuries**. Since 1963, Dr. Benjamin has pioneered in private sports medicine and muscular therapy practice and is the founder and President of the Muscular Therapy Institute in Cambridge, Massachusetts. As an educator and author, he has conducted seminars and workshops across the country, served as an instructor and trainer, and written several books and countless articles. His books include: "*Listen to Your Pain: The Active Person's Guide to Understanding, Identifying, and Treating Pain and Injury*"; "*Are You Tense?: The Benjamin System of Muscular Therapy*", and "*Exercise Without Injury*".

Dr. Benjamin made a profound statement that <u>sacral ligaments torn or scarred by injury can cause the most devastating low-back and leg pain</u>. The sacral ligaments hold and stabilize the sacrum together with the hip joints and pelvis. It is his contention that injuries to the sacral ligaments account for a large majority of low-back, tailbone, and sciatic pain traveling down the leg. Dr. Benjamin has discovered 4 different patterns of pain caused by torn sacral ligaments, especially referred pain which means that you suffered an injury in one area of the body but the pain is felt in another. <u>The evaluation of low-back injuries which are unique for each patient being examined hinges upon understanding referred pain and its patterns.</u> Even though an injury may be the principal cause of pain, lower back pain and pain in the lower extremities usually appear over varying periods of time. Torn sacral ligaments and tissues can be the culprits for the referral of pain down the legs, not a pinched nerve. Pattern 4 is the most intense back pain which does not necessarily involve any leg pain. The patient suffers for so many years with sudden episodes of pain or constant pain and has tried all kinds of drugs, therapy, and even surgery to get relief but to no avail. The patient's quality of life is almost nonexistent and seems irretrievable. Dr. Benjamin's descriptions of these pain patterns can be found in his Internet website <u>www.benbenjamin.com</u>.

My own pattern of pain falls under Category# 2. As a result of repeated injury suffered from prolonged sitting at a desk or in a car, lifting heavy objects, or twisting your body, adhesive scar tissue forms in the sacroiliac and other pelvic ligaments. Over time this weak scar tissue stretches and distends, making the low back more unstable so that repeated injury becomes more likely. For so many years I have felt the lower back pain all the way across it or one side, pain that has made my life so miserable and unpredictable. From time to time the lower back pain tended to move from left to right. During the 1980's I had tried chiropractors such as Dr. John Glaccum in Lilburn, Georgia and Dr. Debra Alsko and her father in Port Charlotte, Florida and osteopaths such as Dr. Morton Brownstein in Sarasota, Florida and even considered the potential of acupuncture for the relief of my back pain and discomfort. During 1987 I decided to build a house in Bradenton, Florida to be nearer to the office in Sarasota. The daily 33-mile drive from North Port Charlotte to Sarasota was a grind that was taking its toll on my lower back and my overall health since I began working for the State of Florida in October 1984. Compounding my daily commute to Sarasota was the fact that most of my sales tax audit assignments were in the Sarasota and Bradenton area. Sometimes I would be driving 50 miles or longer one way to go to various audit sites. From May 1987 until April 1989 I lived in Bradenton near the small town of Oneco off Highway 301 near DeSoto Square Mall. It was during this period of time that I became a patient of David Shue who took care of me for quite some time in 1988. I also found out about Dr. Benjamin and the benefits of prolotherapy (reconstructive proliferant therapy). It is ironic that David Shue was not a proponent of prolotherapy which he felt would not benefit me.

Dr. Benjamin is so passionate about prolotherapy, a medical procedure which involves the injection of proliferants into injured ligaments, muscles, tendons, or joints in order to produce local inflammation. As a result of this intentional inflammation, prolotherapy then triggers the healing process in the body itself when the regenerative process is not activated naturally. Proliferation is defined as the growth or production of cells by multiplication of parts, and prolotherapy uses common chemicals as proliferants to create new tissues by activating the cellular replication in the collagen or connective tissues. The most popular proliferant among those formulas being used in practice that have passed tests for quality assurance and with no side effects is the Ongley solution developed in 1960 by Dr. Milne Ongley. The Ongley solution includes the following ingredients in its formula:

- Dextrose (a pure sugar that your body produces naturally and serves as the main proliferant to stimulate the production of connective tissue; dextrose also aids in the administration of certain medications intraveneously),
- Xylocaine (the numbing medication used by dentists) or a local anesthetic (lidocaine, procaine, or marcaine),
- Glycerine (aids blood clotting), and
- Phenol (a proliferant needed to stop infection).

According to Dr. Benjamin, prolotherapy has been found to be very beneficial in reducing or even eliminating chronic pain in the neck, lower back, chest, shoulders, elbows, wrists, hips, knees, and ankles. Frequently, injuries to joints cause painful scar tissue to form and weaken ligaments or tendons. As new connective tissue develops, its shrinkage tightens and thereby strengthens the affected areas being treated. Weak joints are made stronger through injections that constrict and firm up the tendons and ligaments holding the joints together. Dr. Benjamin stresses the importance of the patient to exercise gingerly and frequently every day to guarantee the effectiveness of the treatments. What I have personally discovered in my own experience and journey is that sets of exercises must be done within a full range of motion for each part of the body to ensure the healing process and new tissue development are successful. Furthermore, success is achieved when patients refrain from early return to stressful activities. Because each person's healing rate varies because of age, health history, strength, flexibility, level of stress, and nutrition, the number of treatments will also vary. Other factors affecting the length of treatments include the part of the body being treated as well as the severity of the injury. I faced the ominous task of trying to find a practitioner in reconstructive proliferant therapy.

I visited the Atlanta metropolitan area in May 1988, and I was totally blown away by the amazing growth and commercial development going on up there since we had relocated to Florida during 1983. Numerous Fortune 500 companies had moved their headquarters to Atlanta, and the business community and the downtown area were booming. It seemed construction and development were under way everywhere in Atlanta. The Sarasota-Bradenton area paled in comparison with its lack of industry and commerce and the vast majority of its population over 65 who are coarse, cold, and uncaring people mostly from the Northeast. I began to realize that my future was not in the area where I was living even though the warmer climate was certainly more tolerable than Atlanta winters. Mother did not want me to leave Florida and relocate to the Atlanta area. She had given Daddy and me the green light to move to Florida in June 1983 despite the fact that her heart and soul were anchored in Atlanta. Mother, who grew up during the Depression years in the Buckhead area, had never lived anywhere else. But she sacrificed her own preferences and emotional ties to Atlanta so that "the boys" could move to where they wanted to live healthier and happier lives.

As a result, I made the fateful decision in April 1989 to relocate to Tallahassee, Florida as the result of a requested transfer to the Department of Revenue's Audit Review Section as a Tax Audit Specialist II. Tallahassee, which is the state capital, is located only 25 miles from the Georgia state line near Thomasville, the *"City of Roses"*, where Tippy had lived for a long time. I can truly appreciate the warm hospitality and the friendliness of the residents of Tallahassee which is more like an extension of South Georgia and a difference between night and day in comparison to Sarasota residents. I shed no tears when I relocated to Tallahassee other than leaving my parents behind in North Port Charlotte. The Department of Revenue in Tallahassee desperately needed experienced auditors in their offices to properly administer and enforce a myriad of revenue laws through the audit staff and collection specialists in the taxpayer service centers and to develop audit policy and procedures for the audit staff to follow in performing audit assignments.

The specialist position afforded me more time and opportunity to explore and finally take advantage of the potential benefits of prolotherapy and at the same time get away from the demanding rigors of auditing. On May 30, 1989 I wrote a letter to Dr. Benjamin stating that "I have just read and studied your articles which appeared in the Fall 1988 and Winter 1989 issues of the *Massage Therapy Journal* pertaining to the causes of lower back pain and various treatments available. A copy of these articles was given to me by Carol Trescott, a physical therapist here in Tallahassee....." On July 11, 1989 I received a reply from Dr. Benjamin at the *Muscular Therapy Institute, Inc.* in the form of 2 articles covering a new treatment for back pain, **Dr. Ongley's "back shot"**. He suggested contacting Dr. Milne Ongley in

Newport Beach, California for referrals in my area. By the grace of God I finally found Dr. Marvin L. Hodson and Dr. David Kudelko, his successor, in Belleair Bluffs, Florida. Dr. Donald R. Furci, whose medical practice is in Sarasota, referred me to Dr. Hodson. Ironically Dr. Furci worked in conjunction with David Shue. I made several trips from Tallahassee to Dr. Hodson's office and followed the following instructions after each surgical procedure:

- Take pain medication with a full glass of water when you first become uncomfortable.
- Use cold packs which may be applied 3 times daily for 20 minutes as needed. You should begin to get relief after the second day.
- Do not participate in any activities involving bending, lifting, raking, mowing, shoveling, sweeping, bowling, or golf or any usual work which causes pain, now or before.
- Try to walk 1 mile per day. (I must have walked a thousand miles.)
- No exercises for 3 weeks following the last treatment.
- For 6 weeks after treatment, avoid lifting any objects over 25 pounds.
- Return to light work when you are able.

In August 1992 I made yet another crucial decision to relocate as a sales tax auditor to the Atlanta Taxpayer Service Center. I knew I was getting back into the game as an auditor out in the field which included overnight travel and "living out of a suitcase" in hotels. I knew I was jumping from "the frying pan into the fire". But the highest salary I ever made in Florida was not quite $30,000 a year, and I was compensated by returning to auditing as a multi-state tax auditor with an additional income of approximately $7,700 a year. After the sale of our house in North Port Charlotte, my parents had joined me in Tallahassee in August 1990 when we built a house in beautiful Killearn Lakes Subdivision with John Long as the contractor. It had been such a difficult choice to leave my parents behind in April 1989, but the distance between us was only going to be 250 miles. Considering the magnitude of my health problems, my parents and I were always close and supportive. However, Mother's health was slowly but surely deteriorating despite my own and my dad's efforts to take care of her. She refused to go to doctors, and her attitude and stubbornness would eventually cost Mother her life.

For me a major consideration was the higher quality of medical treatment and health care facilities available in the Atlanta area. To this moment I feel this decision to relocate to Atlanta in August 1992 ultimately saved my physical and emotional health as well as my life. I had discovered Dr. Ken Knott, a physiatrist, whose medical practice is in Marietta, Georgia. **In the United States, there are over 4,400 physiatrists, or rehabilitation physicians, who are highly trained medical doctors specializing in physical medicine and rehabilitation for the treatment of injuries or diseases that affect the nerves, muscles, and bones.** Specifically, rehabilitation physicians perform the following medical procedures in order to restore the body's mobility and flexibility:

- **Diagnose the cause and symptoms of pain for proper non-surgical treatment which includes the entire body, not just the area of concern.**
- **Regain the maximum function that has been lost through injury, illness or disability.**
- **Explain your health problems as well as a treatment and prevention plan managed through the collaborative efforts of other health care professionals such as neurologists, orthopedic surgeons, and physical therapists.**

A rehabilitation physician concentrates upon the establishment of an in-depth program for the treatment of any disability caused by an injury or illness, including a team of health care professionals. This program includes the restoration of the patient's quality of life and active lifestyle after the injury or disease which has been treated without resorting to surgery. The treatment plan can also be carried out by the patients themselves. These health care professionals possess extensive medical experience and knowledge which makes them indispensable in treating future health issues throughout a person's lifetime, if necessary.

What made Dr. Knott so unique and incredibly successful with the treatment of my injured back and left hip was his **integration of prolotherapy into the healing process. The combination of physiatry and prolotherapy had made the dramatic difference in strengthening and rehabilitating my injured lower back and sacral ligaments.** I have undergone over 20 surgical procedures using prolotherapy. During some of these injections I had to endure excruciating pain in my spine and joints. But the pain and discomfort gradually went away after applying ice packs and walking. Dr. Knott firmly believes in exercise with weights and also Pilates or other physical fitness regimens during these treatments. When I was sideswiped by another vehicle in September 2004, my right hip was injured. Dr. Knott repaired my injured right hip with prolotherapy, and fortunately Liberty Mutual Insurance, my insurance carrier at the time of the accident, covered my medical expenses. During 2009 I began to experience pain and discomfort as well as stiffness in my left knee which was injured in the 1981 automobile accident. Dr. Knott successfully treated the knee with prolotherapy with only 3 visits which strengthened and alleviated the inflammation of the knee joint diagnosed as chronic malacia.

I can never overemphasize the importance of taking vitamin and mineral supplements not just for overall health and fitness but also during the healing process of medical treatment like prolotherapy or surgery. My dad urged me to begin taking vitamin supplements which he himself had been taking. Everyone's dietary needs, however, are different based upon a number of factors including age, lifestyle, diet, stress, medications, and others. As the result of my titanic struggles with other health problems and suffering with the back and hip injuries, I have discovered and adhered to **4 important and essential principles for healthy living: 1) eating healthy and nutritious foods; 2) daily exercise; 3) getting plenty of sleep and rest, and 4) the incorporation of the following vitamins and minerals into my diet**:

Vitamin C

According to *MedlinePlus Medical Encyclopedia [March 21, 2017]*, Vitamin C is an antioxidant that dissolves in water and the body needs it to grow or regenerate tissues. This vitamin literally becomes a part of protein for the formation of skin, ligaments, teeth, bones, and blood vessels and for the healing of injuries with the formation of scar tissue.

I take 5,000 mg of Vitamin C because you have to take the vitamin or eat foods rich in Vitamin C on a daily basis in order to replenish it every day.

Vitamin E

In his Internet website *DrWeil.com [March 21, 2017]*, Vitamin E is described as a powerful antioxidant that has no known side effects and is essential in maintaining heart health, including red blood cell reproduction and cardiac muscle. This vitamin may promote immune health, prevent cancer, slow down the effects of Alzheimer's Disease, and prevent damage to the eyes caused by diabetes. In addition, Vitamin E is essential in building up sources of Vitamin A, Vitamin K, iron, and selenium.

I personally take 800 IU of Vitamin E each day.

CoEnzyme Q10

In his Internet website *DrWeil.com [March 21, 2017]*, Dr. Weil discusses the benefits of **Coenzyme Q10 (CoQ10)** which is described as a natural antioxidant found in every cell of the body and can be taken as a very safe supplement or contained in many foods. CoQ10 plays a vital role in metabolism in the generation of energy within cells, especially in such organs as the kidneys, liver, and heart which have high demands for energy. This vitamin promotes heart health and circulation as well as the function of heart muscle.

<u>Believe me, CoEnzymeQ10 is one amazing vitamin supplement. I myself take 400 mg per day.</u>

Cordyceps Sinensis Mushroom Extract

Cordyceps (*Cordyceps sinensis, Sphaeria sinensis*) is a mushroom fungus found on the bodies of caterpillars living in China. Pursuant to Dr. Mark Stengler's *Natural Healing Library (2013)*, clinical research has proven that *Cordyceps* restores the immune function and improves the condition of patients with the following serious diseases or health problems:

- Asthma
- Chronic bronchitis
- Emphysema
- Heart disease

- Cancer
- Adrenal glands (energy production, stamina, and endurance)
- Chronic fatigue
- Kidney function
- Hepatitis B
- Diabetes

Please check out Dr. Stengler's book *Natural Healing Library* for additional information.

Glutathione

In his Internet website *[March 21, 2017]*, Dr. Mark Hyman explains that glutathione is a recycler of antioxidants that not only is a relatively unknown vitamin but also is an uncomplicated molecule of proteins with the key to unlock a healthy body and stop disease dead in its tracks. Glutathione, which is produced in the human body, can unfortunately be exhausted as the result of improper nutrition, old age, poor air quality, stressful lifestyles, prescription drugs, infections, poisons, and radiation therapy. Sickness, age, or poor physical health generally is indicative of a glutathione deficiency. As a matter of fact, studies have uncovered that the levels of this vitamin vary greatly with the age of patients. The highest level is in healthy young people, while the lowest level was found in the elderly. Obviously, the production and preservation of high levels of glutathione in the body is imperative to recover from almost any and all serious diseases much less to stay healthy and to optimize performance. According to Dr. Hyman, this molecule can literally protect the human body from cancer, heart disease, and dementia as well as fight infections and reverse the process of aging. Exercise such as aerobics, walking, jogging, or playing your favorite sports, eating foods containing glutathione, and taking supplements are ways to increase the supply of glutathione in the body. **I personally take 400 mg of glutathione every day.**

In addition, Dr. Hyman emphasizes the importance and benefits of the following vitamin supplements:

- **N-acetyl-cysteine (NAC).** This supplement is very beneficial in the treatment of asthma sufferers and lung diseases. **I personally take**

> 1,200 mg every day because I suffer with chronic bronchiectasis, a form of COPD.

- **Alpha lipoic acid.** Only glutathione is more important than this particular compound which the body produces in our cells. Alpha lipoic acid generates energy, regulates blood sugar, and promotes brain health, but its supply is often exhausted as the result of the stress of life. **(I personally take 1,200 mg every day as a supplement to my diet.)**
- **Selenium.** This important mineral helps the body recycle and produce more glutathione.
- **Vitamin C and Vitamin E as well as other antioxidants** team up to recycle glutathione.

For more information about the nature and substance of glutathione and these other important vitamins, please refer to Dr. Mark Hyman's website on the Internet.

Zinc

According to *WebMD.com* *[March 21, 2017]*, small amounts of zinc are essential to promote human health, including but not limited to the following health problems:

- Maintain and promote the immune system
- Treat the common cold, chronic ear and lower respiratory infections, and viruses
- Accelerate the healing of wounds and blood clotting
- Use for the treatment of eye diseases such as macular degeneration and for night blindness and cataracts because of high concentrations of zinc in the eye
- Treat major depression, digestive problems, Type 2 diabetes, thyroid function, high blood pressure, AIDS, tinnitus, osteoporosis, rheumatoid arthritis, Alzheimer's Disease, skin conditions, and serious head trauma.

Dietary supplements can be taken for zinc deficiency. Furthermore, a change in diet containing sufficient levels of zinc should include food products such as meat, seafood, milk and cheese, nuts, beans, and whole grains.

Potassium

Under *WebMD.com's* Internet website *[March 21, 2017]*, it is stated that the mineral potassium is so critical for the proper functioning of the heart, kidneys, and other important organs. Because so many people do not eat a healthy diet, they may have a deficiency of potassium and are susceptible to high blood pressure, heart disease, stroke, arthritis, cancer, and digestive disorders. A potassium deficiency requires a better diet or supplements for prevention or treatment. Smoking, substance abuse, Crohn's Disease, athletic competition, certain medications, eating disorders, and physically demanding work can be detrimental to the body's supply of potassium.

Final Note: After several discussions with doctors, chiropractors, neurosurgeons, physical therapists, pain management specialists, neuromuscular massage therapists, and even dentists, it is alarming to me that there tends to be a lack of communication and collaboration among fellow health care professionals to work together for the benefit of the patients under their care. The interaction of all health care professionals and the exchange of ideas and philosophies are not only invaluable for health care practitioners themselves but also for the success of medical treatments and the overall health and healing of the patients under their care.

Never underestimate the will power and resolve of your adversaries, but then never underestimate the might and power of God who defeats and subdues your Goliaths.

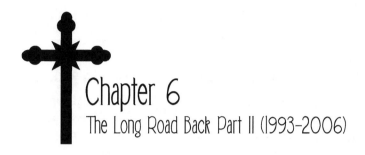

Chapter 6
The Long Road Back Part II (1993-2006)

Christopher Reeve once said that "[a] hero is an ordinary individual who finds the strength to persevere and endure in spite of overwhelming obstacles." I believe that the actor who portrayed Superman in the movies could have had me in mind when he made this statement. I began to feel that my physical problems and difficulties were insurmountable. I still thank God for my parents who constantly prayed for me and gave me daily support and encouragement which I so desperately needed each day to survive my "roller coaster" life.

In the late 1980's, when I lived in Tallahassee, I began to suffer with facial pain, headaches, teeth pain, soreness in my jaw, and neck and shoulder pain, symptoms I had not experienced before. In the summer of 1980 I had been kicked in the face during a softball tournament when I was sliding into 2nd base and the infielder leaped to catch the throw from the outfield. I remember that I had suffered my 3rd concussion, and I was unable to open my mouth wide for 2 or 3 days because of a locked jaw, but I never did go to a doctor for examination of my injury. I was 30 years old at the time, and I never gave it a thought that this was going to be the tragic continuation of the series of serious, life-changing injuries. A year later, my face apparently smashed into the steering wheel and two of my front teeth were badly chipped in the automobile accident in October 1981. I do not recall my face hitting anything, so crushing and debilitating was the blow to my head when I was propelled into the windshield upon impact that caused the 4th concussion of my lifetime and hopefully my last. I told Dr. Knott about the diagnosis of TMJ or TMD [temporomandibular joint dysfunction] by Dr. Hughes. Dr. Knott did treat me for TMD, but it was his professional opinion that Dr. Hughes was the best specialist and medical internist available to address the medical treatment of TMD. Dr. Knott was right.

On its Internet website, *WebMD.com [March 21, 2017]* explains that the temporomandibular joint controls the movement of the jaw and the muscles in the face so that a person can talk, chew, and yawn. The dysfunction of the jaw and facial muscles is called temporomandibular disorder (TMD). **The causes of TMD still remain unknown. However, dentists maintain that injured or weakened muscles within the jaw or damage to the soft disc between the ball and socket of the joint itself often cause severe pain or discomfort which can be temporary or long-lasting. TMD, it is believed, is attributable to a sharp blow to the face or jaw joint or a whiplash injury to the muscles controlling the movement of the head and neck. I have experienced both. Job stress, arthritis, and bruxing or clinching your teeth can also contribute to TMD by causing pressure upon the movements of the jaw joint and tightening the jaw and facial muscles.**

According to *WebMD.com [March 21, 2017]*, the dentist will ask a patient about his or her health history and examine the jaw as well as the face and neck to verify the presence and severity of TMD. Oddly enough, women are more likely to suffer with TMD than men, and TMD usually afflicts young people between 20 and 40. Before taking X-rays or using other diagnostic tests such as a MRI and CT scans, the dentist will check for the common symptoms which could affect only one or both sides of the face and include but are not limited to the following:

- Pain or sensitivity in the face, jaw joint, neck, and shoulders which results in headaches, neck aches, tinnitus, or earaches (I suffered with intense headaches in the middle of my forehead, tenderness in my jaw joint, and pain going all the way down from my neck to my lower back.)
- Tooth decay, teeth pain, and gingivitis (I suffered with teeth pain and sensitivity in my gums.)
- Sinusitis or hearing problems (I suffer with acute sinusitis.)
- Arthritis
- Difficulty in opening up your mouth wide, including the jaw freezing in position whether or not the mouth is open; clicking, snapping, or grinding noises inside the jaw, including whenever chewing food
- Difficulty chewing food or experiencing discomfort with the bite of the upper and lower teeth
- Dizziness

The dentist can also discuss with the patient the following traditional treatments for TMD:

- **Medications.**
- **A splint or night guard.**
- **Dental work, including conferring with an orthodontist.**

Doctors can suggest available home remedies listed below that patients can use to help relieve TMD symptoms:

- Take over-the-counter pain and anti-inflammatory medications.
- Apply moist heat or cold packs. This treatment helped with my pain and discomfort temporarily.
- The dentist or physical therapist may recommend simple jaw stretches, along with holding a warm compress to the side of your face for about 5 minutes. Paula Parcheta, a neuromuscular therapist, taught me the "tongue roll" inside my mouth which does relax the jaw and facial muscles affected by TMD.
- Eat soft foods.
- Minimize yawning and chewing and do not chew gum or ice. In addition, by keeping the lower and upper teeth apart often or putting the tongue between the teeth, jaw and facial muscles will relax which should alleviate the pain and discomfort.
- Always try to maintain good posture.
- Never rest your chin on your hand or hold the telephone between your shoulder and ear.
- Consider physical or neuromuscular massage therapy. Both therapies have helped me immensely with the pain and discomfort caused by TMD.

A dentist may talk with patients about the following possibilities for other treatments:

- **Transcutaneous electrical nerve stimulation (TENS).**
- **Ultrasound.**
- **Trigger-point injections for pain relief.**

- **Radio wave therapy.**
- **Low-level laser therapy.**

Surgery is also an option for further care and treatment. An oral surgeon specializes in surgery involving the entire face, mouth, and jaw. Depending upon the nature and severity of the jaw problem, the following types of surgery can be performed for TMD:

- **Arthrocentesis**
- **Arthroscopy**
- **Open-joint surgery**

For further discussion and information concerning the treatment options for TMD, please refer to the Internet website for *WebMD.com*.

According to *Dr. Michael Westman [March 21, 2017]*, a dentist in Racine, Wisconsin, the symptoms of TMD frequently emerge from the loss of a permanent tooth and force the surrounding teeth to literally move and close the gap created by the missing tooth. This unnatural shift in the teeth, in turn, causes the misalignment of your natural bite which will require special dental work to correct. That is exactly what happened to me when I had 2 molars pulled in my lower left jaw as the result of an abscess and a cracked tooth, coupled with blows to my face and head caused by sports injuries and the automobile accident in October 1981. Dr. Westman describes many popular options involving dental implants for the treatment of TMD to address the pain which can be minor or severe. He explains that traditional bridge or partial denture can be used to replace gaps and spaces in the teeth. However, the dentist plays a major role in providing care and maintenance that are required for these two options. A dental implant is a permanent option that fits in with your regular dental routine easily and, more importantly, helps correct a patient's bite to relieve the TMD discomfort.

On its Internet website, *WebMD.com [March 21, 2017]* describes in detail the dental implant procedure that is designed and customized for each patient's unique treatment plan for his or her specific needs. Highly trained and experienced health care professionals specializing in oral surgery and curative dentistry develop the most suitable treatment plan containing the best implant option for the patient. On January 11, 1993 I underwent dental implant surgery to correct my bite and thereby relieve my TMD symptoms by replacing 2 back molars in my lower jaw. Simultaneously, I regularly had neuromuscular massage therapy to complement and maintain the success and integrity of the implant surgery. I also began to work out with weights at the gym under the scrutiny of Dr. Knott who was still involved in the care of my lower back. Neuromuscular massage therapy was continuing to be beneficial to my overall health and emotional well-being as I was working under tremendous pressure and stress for the State of Florida as a tax auditor.

But the medical treatment of concussions and brain injuries is an entirely different matter. After suffering at least 4 concussions (2 severe) and several other head injuries during my lifetime, I wish I had had the *Brain Injury Association of America* at the time to explain the nature and symptoms of a mild traumatic brain injury. In its *Report to Congress on Mild Traumatic Brain Injury in the United States*, the *Centers for Disease Control* defined the term mild traumatic brain injury: an injury caused from blunt trauma to the head, which is transmitted to the brain with the mechanical force of the impact, and can result in one or more of the following side effects or physical reactions:

- Confusion, disorientation, or impaired consciousness;
- Amnesia around the time of injury;
- Seizures acutely following head injury;
- Loss of consciousness lasting 30 minutes or less (Believe it or not, a brain injury does not necessarily cause unconsciousness).

The damage caused by the *invisible* mild brain injury sometimes adversely affects the ability of victims to successfully return to their lives by changing their thinking patterns and memory. This experience happened to me with muddled thinking and short memory loss suffered from such *mild brain injuries*. The *American Psychological Association* highly recommends the consideration of neuropsychological evaluations when the functional effects of a mild brain injury should be tested and verified. These evaluations are performed whenever the doctors suspect some type of brain dysfunction. You can read more about neuropsychological evaluations and brain injury from the *American Psychological Association*. In addition, more recent and more complicated imaging technologies that can possibly aid in diagnosis and treatment by capturing the damage caused by a mild brain injury include the following:

- Positron Emission Tomography (PET Scan)
- Single Photon Emission Computerized Tomography
- Functional Magnetic Resonance Imaging
- Diffuse Tensor Imaging

Paramount to the recovery process is educating and informing the family and friends of the victims of the invisible changes caused by a brain injury. This education and awareness is also very important for the victim as well. Listed below are basic symptoms for family and friends to be aware of:

Early Symptoms:

- Headaches
- Dizzy spells or loss of equilibrium
- Confusion
- Nausea with or without memory loss or vomiting

Later Symptoms:

- Constant but minor headache
- Vertigo
- Short attention span and lack of concentration
- Unusual fatigue
- Extreme sensitivity to bright light or vision difficulties
- Extreme sensitivity to loud noises; tinnitus
- Anxiety and depression
- Irritable and easily frustrated state of mind

It is extremely difficult to make the distinction between a concussion and a mild brain injury. Brain injuries can consist of a concussion and a mild, moderate, and severe brain injury. **A concussion is defined as a traumatic physical injury to the brain that disrupts and causes a change in its normal function affecting physical or cognitive abilities. Blows to the head or a severe whiplash are major causes of concussions which do not necessarily result in a loss of consciousness.** If you suspect you have suffered a mild brain injury, please contact a health care professional versed in the diagnosis and treatment of a brain injury. Also, please contact the *Brain Injury Association* in your state. State *Brain Injury Associations* will have information to share and can connect you with support groups, programs, and health care professionals who understand the injury. The *American Academy of Neurology (AAN)* and the *Brain Injury Association (BIA)* have developed guidelines for classifying the different types of concussions.

As I said before, Mother's life ended tragically in September 1993 when she fell down the steps in the garage of the Stockbridge, Georgia house during a visit to see me. The fall had shattered her left hip so badly that the surgeons could nothing to save her hip or her life. It took many, many years for me to deal and cope with the death of my beloved mother on December 4, 1993. Her death created a void in my life that I have never filled since her departure. Mother was always my best friend, guide, mentor, extraordinary prayer warrior, and confidante. At that time Dr. C. R. Hill was the Senior Pastor at McDonough First United Methodist Church where Daddy and I were members. Dr. Hill wrote this beautiful epitaph for my mother's funeral service bulletin and as a keepsake for my father, family members, and me which I have since shared with many, many grieving people over the years:

Sailing with the Evening Tide

"I've taken sail with the evening tide,
Over the waning moonlit sea.
I am crossing over to the other side,
Where Jesus awaits to welcome me.

I know my leaving will cause you pain,
But your sorrow is for season brief.
You will find joy in hope for I'll see you again,
While from my suffering I've been granted relief.

I've journeyed on to my heavenly home,
Where my inheritance has forever been.
Now by God's grace and love you will carry on,
Until in His presence we'll be together again.

Hold fast the faith that we cherished below,
That served [as] a compass and guide and chart,
And remember the love that gave us life,
Then hold steady God's course in your heart.

The days of earth are fleeting at best,
They are given for faith to mature,
Those who through their trials shall stand the test.
Will taste of life in Jesus secure."

IN MEMORY OF VIRGINIA NELSON HIME
12/7/1993

After the loss of my mother, Daddy felt the same way I did about being miles apart, and it came to no surprise that we decided he should move into the Stockbridge house to live with me so that he would not be living alone in Tallahassee 250 miles away. At that point in time, my dad was 75 years old and had been retired 10 years from Fulton Supply Company.

The great and challenging adjustment for me was conducting sales and corporate income tax audits away from home and living "out of a suitcase" in hotel rooms. But to tell the truth, I adjusted well to being on the road. I consider the job of tax auditor to be one of the toughest jobs in auditing and accounting. A tax auditor has to wear so many "hats" in this line of work—accountant, computer analyst, Perry Mason, secretary, writer, Columbo, negotiator, diplomat, and credit manager. Unfortunately, some auditors treated me as if I had no business being in their office. I had "earned my stripes" after working out in the field for 5 years in Sarasota and serving as a Tax Audit Specialist in Audit Review for 3 years. But I was snubbed by a few because I had been an in-state sales tax auditor who audited mostly small "mom and pop" businesses. I was now working in Multi-State Audits where the stakes were much higher since we audited the Fortune 500 companies located in the Southeast who were conducting business in Florida.

At the time, I had to work under difficult circumstances because I was suffering so much with TMJ pain and discomfort as well as back pain. Before we purchased the Stockbridge house on March 4, 1993, I had been renting a home for 5 months in nearby Jonesboro from a landlord who was unscrupulous and devious to deal with. The landlord would eventually and falsely accuse me of deliberating flooding his basement twice which knocked out the furnace. The year 1992 was one of the wettest in the history of Atlanta, and rotted out gutters on the house did not help the situation either. When flooding knocked out the furnace the second time, the temperature inside the house dropped to 44 degrees, and I had to go to a local hotel to stay warm for the night.

Enough was enough. The great tragedy of this predicament was the painful decision as to whether or not to "break the lease" which was for the usual 12 months in duration. I began to search frantically to find another place to live without having any "game plan" to make wise decisions about possibly purchasing a home. I had planned to rent a house for at least 2 years before I made the decision on where to live and to settle down. I had not lived in the Atlanta area since July 1983, and a lot had changed with the growth and the development of my hometown with the influx of big business and its work force. When I was growing up in East Point, the population of Atlanta was a mere 200,000. Another factor was the booming housing market at that time, and houses were being snatched up left and right. Realtors were helping me to find a house in Stockbridge, and I had finally found a house that was ideal, a 3 bedroom, 2 bath house with a large yard. I prepared to present an escrow check to the sales agent at the subdivision, and the moment I did I was told that someone else had beaten me to his office to buy this particular house. I told the sales agent I was bringing a deposit, and he betrayed me. Because of the time constraints facing me with "breaking the lease" on the rental house, I was saddled with purchasing the last available house on a sloped corner lot. This house would prove to be Mother's undoing. The slope of the lot required building the house with a crawl space and steps to the front porch and to the side door to the garage. We lived in Stockbridge from 1993 until Christmas 2001 when we had to move to the Roswell area just before our office was later relocated to Marietta from College Park near the Atlanta Airport in June 2002. I strongly felt we both needed a change of scenery because of the tragedy that had occurred inside that house and the loss of our first Schnauzer to colon cancer.

And, of course, I had to adapt and learn how to sleep in a hotel room on the road in "foreign" locales where I knew absolutely no one and the taxpayers I was auditing did not want me there in the first place. I was the infamous and notorious "tax man". I soon realized that I would have to prove myself in the eyes of both the audit staff and the taxpayers, and I was so bound and determined that I belonged there by proving myself through my performance out in the field and the use of my technical knowledge of Florida tax laws and statutes. It was puzzling to me that I noticed right away the audit staff was so poorly versed in the interpretation and application of the Florida sales tax rules and statutes.

I do not know how to explain it, but tax auditors are much like police officers and firemen in that we have joined a fraternity that lasts long after we work for the State of Florida. We are entrusted with the duty and responsibility of auditing the accounting records and documents for compliance and enforcement of Florida tax laws and statutes. Tackling difficult taxpayers who have enormous resources at their disposal and defending our positions on tax and legal issues against high price lawyers and accounting firms require auditors to pull together and pool our own resources of knowledge and experience to represent the State of Florida's interests. But at the same time we have to be fair and equitable with the taxpayers in interpreting and applying Florida tax laws. At times I felt like I was the reincarnation of David fighting Goliath again and again whenever I had to confront large taxpayers at their place of business. Auditors have to learn how to adjust and adapt to hostile audit environments, uncooperative taxpayer personnel, voluminous records, sometimes dusty and dirty working conditions in warehouses or storage facilities, and deadlines to complete audit assignments. Our job as auditors is extremely negative in nature with little or no positive reinforcement. Yet tax auditors are civil servants of the public who indeed pay our salaries through the taxes the public pays whenever a taxable transaction occurs in Florida, whether it be paying for a hotel room, going out to eat at a restaurant, buying gasoline, going to Disney World, enjoying the beach, or buying groceries. To me this has always been an awesome responsibility that we have been entrusted with to serve the public and the 20,000,000 citizens of Florida. As Sir Winston Churchill once said, "**the price of greatness is responsibility**".

In **Colossians, Chapter 3 [New King James Version]**, I found in the Bible the heart of my philosophy of working for a living that I had come to live by:

"²³ **And whatever you do, do it heartily, as to the Lord
and not to men, ²⁴ knowing that from the Lord you will
receive the reward of the inheritance; for you serve the
Lord Christ."**

Whenever I deal with people, either friend or foe, I remember the famous
scripture in the Bible that is contained in **Matthew 7, Verse 12 [New King
James Version]**—

"¹² **Therefore, whatever you want men to do to you, do
also to them, for this is the Law and the Prophets." The
Golden Rule.**

It was a sworn oath for me that I treat others the way I want them to
treat me in return. My parents had brought me up in that way in a loving
Christian environment.

My dad and I had become closer and closer after Mother's untimely
death. As a result, it was not a difficult adjustment for us to live together.
I am forever indebted and grateful to my mother and father who were
compassionate and gracious enough to follow me everywhere I moved to after
the tragic automobile accident in October 1981. Some friends questioned
why my parents were following me around from one place to another. No
one knew about the nature and seriousness of the health problems I was
plagued and suffering with except my parents. Without a wife and a family of
my own to take care of me, Mother and Daddy were, in effect, my caregivers
and sole support. Without them I would have never survived spiritually and
emotionally, much less physically.

From December 1993 until the beginning of 2001, my dad was in good
health and sharp as a tack mentally. He had a wealth of knowledge about the
stock market and the economy. Daddy made the decisions about investments
by reading about and studying the stock market in such magazines as
Kiplinger's, The Bottom Line, Consumer Reports, and *Money Magazine* and by
following such experts as Louis Rukeyser, Frank Cappiello, Gail Dudack,
Carter Randall, Julius Westheimer, and Martin Zweig on *Wall Street Week.*
I truly miss Daddy's acumen and wisdom as I do Mother's wit, sense of
humor, positive attitude, prayers, and common sense advice. Daddy and

I had been working out together at the health clubs as well as jogging and working out on the basketball court ever since 1968, and we both ate well to stay healthy. My travel schedule often interrupted my routines with him. Later Daddy would decide to go with me on audit trips so that he would not be left alone. He always supported me when I had to work so many hours on audit assignments. Cooking meals, washing clothes, dusting and cleaning the house, going to the grocery store, walking the dog. With my dad's help and encouragement, I excelled in my audit work. I won the 1997 *Davis Productivity Award* for my audit field work involving a huge corporation.

My dad and I resumed sailing on our *Hunter18.5* at Lake Sinclair near Eatonton and Jackson Lake in Butts County. The dogs always enjoyed going out on the sailboat. I became a Big Brother again in 1997 when I was assigned to Karl Lee Martin who was 5 years old and lived not too far from us. A natural lefthander, Karl excelled in the bowling alley where he became a good bowler. He loved to play video games and ride go-carts, and he eventually played Little League baseball. Karl and Randy Jones, the other boy I was assigned to be a Big Brother for, both enjoyed boating, especially running and steering the boat motor. Being a mentor and bringing joy and happiness to a fatherless boy brought me such great satisfaction and peace and so it did for my parents, too. God gave me the wisdom and guidance to be a surrogate father by making me realize that I myself could enjoy being a boy again. When we had to relocate to the north side of town, I had to discontinue my relationship with Karl as a Big Brother. Sailing on Jackson Lake came to an abrupt halt during the summer of 2001. I can honestly say it was one of the greatest sailing experiences I have ever had, including even those on Lake Lanier and Lake Hartwell.

During 1997 I began to experience serious stomach problems, and I also was suffering with mysterious chest pains. Of course, I had had serious lung problems since March 1966, and chest discomfort seemed to be my constant companion. My chest discomfort became so severe that my doctor ordered a heart catherization at Southern Regional Hospital in Jonesboro on February 26, 1998. The test results were negative although they showed that I did have a weak heart. I can point to the inability of being unable to run and work out effectively as the culprit. In the hospital a nurse commented that my stomach and chest discomfort might be linked to acid reflux, and she recommended for me to undergo yet another upper GI series. Here again I was dealing with stomach issues. Doctors told me that acid reflux can cause chest pains which mimic the symptoms of a heart attack. Daddy had suffered for years with ulcers and a neck injury that caused him such great pain and suffering. Mother also had stomach problems, including irritated bowel syndrome which I inherited from her and my dad. I have been prescribed Protonics, Nexium, Prevacid, Aciphex, and Dexilant for acid reflux which has made my life so miserable at times. Change of diet, drinking water, plus raising the head of the bed, has helped me immensely along with medication.

But my dad was not so lucky with his stomach, especially later in taking medications. For years he had suffered so much with ulcers and possibly acid reflux. I began to notice that Daddy was having trouble hearing me even when he was sitting next to me in the car. We eventually went to an audiologist who determined that indeed he had hearing loss. Daddy needed hearing aids for each ear. The cost of a hearing aid ranges anywhere from $800 up to $5,000. What is staggering is **Medicare does not cover the purchase of such health care products**. Most of us are totally unaware that **in most circumstances Medicare does not cover certain health care services, including room and meals, provided by nursing homes and especially assisted living facilities.** The cost of an assisted living facility can run over $5,000 per month which is self-pay, i.e., it comes out of your pocket. The cost of nursing home care is well over $72,000 a year.

That is why it was so crucial to have someone who "knows the ropes" and specializes in understanding and working with the program benefits, policies and procedures, guidelines, and limitations of Medicare and Medicaid for health care services and medical treatment. In September 1993 Marilyn Peskin-Kaufman first helped Daddy and me to take care of my mother after she had broken her hip and was placed in a nursing home. Marilyn would be so instrumental in orchestrating and coordinating the health care of my mother in 1993 and later on for my father's health care from 2001 through 2003. After Marilyn was seriously injured in an automobile accident, she decided to retire early. Mandy Merkel eventually took her place to oversee my dad's health care and well-being and was such a great advisor as the founder and owner of *Senior Resource Consulting.* Mandy's claim to fame is the use of her hands in the Palmolive dish detergent TV commercials. But her true value is in her compassionate dedication to elderly health care. Mandy has worked in the rehabilitation and long-term care industry for more than 20 years, and she began her career as Director of Outpatient Services for the rehabilitation unit of a hospital in Atlanta. Later she served as Regional Director of Operations for SunDance Rehabilitation Corporation. In her own words, *"Senior Resource Consulting* was formed in response to the growing and critical need of today's elderly population and their families. We are dedicated to empowering seniors and their adult children to have more control over the complex process of finding appropriate senior housing. With more than 20 years of experience in the long-term care arena, we bring valuable insights and offer independent advice on the array of senior housing options to be considered....In working with clients, we take a hands-on approach, doing something we can to guide seniors and their families through a difficult, and often overwhelming, transition process. We perform many tasks that, due to time or distance, may not be possible for family members to handle on their own. Our services range from a detailed analysis of current health and housing status, and assessment of the appropriate level of housing, to specific recommendations for placement, based on availability and on-site visits, if desired. We also offer elder mediation to resolve conflicts in a range of situations among all concerned parties, and ongoing care management regarding medication, treatment, and visitation." Without the assistance of Marilyn and Mandy, I would not have survived in taking care of my dad for over 4 years.

Doctors had been treating Daddy for an inner ear infection. He had been complaining to me and the doctors that he was having problems with his equilibrium and balance when he was walking. Daddy felt like he was going to fall down most of the time. He also had great difficulty getting out of a chair, and I would have to help him get up. I began to notice a slight tremor in his right hand. These physical problems are classic symptoms of *Parkinson's Disease,* another silent killer. According to the *American Parkinson Disease Association,* Parkinson's is a chronic progressive neurological disease that attacks a small area of nerve cells in the brain called neurons. The tragedy and mercilessness of Parkinson's Disease is its destruction of these neurons which normally produce dopamine. This chemical compound transmits signals within the areas of the brain that coordinate smooth and balanced muscle movement if not impaired by disease or injury. Other areas of the brain governing non-motor functions can also be affected by Parkinson's Disease. As a result, body movements and other functions are affected by the symptoms of Parkinson's Disease. Unfortunately, it is still unknown what causes these cells to die.

In its Internet website, *American Parkinson Disease Association* states that when a person in the age range of 21 to 40 is diagnosed with Parkinson's Disease, it is called *young or early onset Parkinson's Disease.* Michael J. Fox is probably the most famous young patient who was diagnosed with young or early onset Parkinson's Disease in 1991 at the age of 30 years old. Fox, the talented Hollywood actor, did not disclose his illness to the general public for another 7 years. He has survived the ravages of Parkinson's Disease for 25 years and counting. From that point on, Fox committed himself to campaign for increased Parkinson's research. In January 2000 he decided to retire from the TV program *Spin City* which was in its fourth season and had reached 100 episodes. The weekly TV show had become too demanding for Fox. Later that year he launched *The Michael J. Fox Foundation for Parkinson's Research,* which the *New York Times* has called "the most credible voice on Parkinson's research in the world." Today the Foundation has become the world's largest nonprofit source of funding of Parkinson's drug research, and the Foundation has been the spearhead to find the cure for Parkinson's Disease. Michael J. Fox has gained widespread admiration and respect for his tenacious work as a patient advocate.

Per the *American Parkinson Disease Association,* generally speaking, a young person usually tends to tolerate the unrelenting progression and symptoms of Parkinson's Disease such as memory loss, confusion, and balance difficulties, mainly because younger people tend to have fewer health problems. Nevertheless, a young person as well as his or her family still have to face the medical, psychological, and social challenges of contending with Parkinson's Disease. The most commonly prescribed medication for Parkinson's Disease is *levodopa* which temporarily restores the action of dopamine in the brain. Unfortunately, young people stricken with Parkinson's Disease often have had more problems with involuntary movements because of taking *levadopa,* and so these young onset patients are usually prescribed medications other than *levodopa* for initial treatment. On its Internet website the *MayoClinic.org* commented that each person's symptoms and warning signs of Parkinson's Disease are unique and different. Sometimes these warning signs can be so mild they are ignored. Symptoms frequently start on just one side of the body where the effects are worse on that particular side, even though the symptoms of the disease will eventually afflict both sides of the body. The following are typical signs and symptoms of Parkinson's Disease:

- **Tremor.** A common trait of Parkinson's Disease is the hand or fingers shaking, especially when the hand is at rest. My father had such a tremor.
- **Slowed movement.** As time goes by, Parkinson's Disease restricts and slows down body movements which can make even the simplest tasks more difficult and so tedious. My father suffered with the difficulty of getting out of a chair, and he also dragged or shuffled his feet so he could make his steps shorter when walking and maintaining his balance.
- **Stiff muscles.** Muscles may become stiff in any part of the body, a debilitating and painful condition which can limit your range of motion.
- **Impaired posture and loss of equilibrium.** The patient has stooped posture or suffers with balance problems caused by Parkinson's Disease. In addition, I notice my father had bent legs whenever he walked.
- **Loss of unconscious movements.** Parkinson's Disease may hinder a patient's ability to blink, smile, or swing the arms when walking.
- **Speech changes.** Parkinson's Disease can adversely affect a person's speech which can become slurred or soft or quick in tone.
- **Writing changes.** A person can experience difficulty in writing, and your writing may appear small.

According to the *American Parkinson Disease Association*, the non-motor symptoms of Parkinson's Disease include but are not limited to the following:

- Mood swings, especially depression which my father experienced
- Sleep disorders or difficulty sleeping
- Changes in thinking
- Problems with low blood pressure, bowel and bladder function, and sweating
- Skin problems

The *American Parkinson Disease Association* emphasizes that every symptom listed does not have to be present to consider and confirm the diagnosis of Parkinson's Disease. For example, a tremor in a person's hand does not prove that he or she has Parkinson's Disease nor does a person have to have a tremor. The cause of Parkinson's Disease is not yet known, and clinical research concentrates upon the effects of genetic, hereditary, environmental, and external factors. Yet no cure or ways to prevent the disease have been discovered. It is sometimes called 'the older person's' disease because it generally afflicts people over the age of 60. Studies show that slightly more men than women tend to contract Parkinson's Disease. Nevertheless, most patients that suffer with Parkinson's Disease can still enjoy active and rewarding lives if neurologists can identify the symptoms of this disease and prescribe the proper medical treatment. My dad admitted to me later that he had made a big mistake to stop working out at the health club in 2000. He had been working out with me since 1968, but at that point in time he was 82 years old. Daddy felt that he might be hurting himself by lifting weights and exercising.

If someone suspects he or she has Parkinson's Disease, a neurologist who is specially trained to diagnose and treat conditions of the brain and nervous system should be consulted. Some neurologists concentrate entirely in working with Parkinson's Disease patients, including those with symptoms of early onset Parkinson's Disease. It has been estimated that roughly 1,500,000 Americans suffer with Parkinson's Disease, and 60,000 new cases are discovered every year. The main objective of performing any additional testing for Parkinson's Disease is to eliminate other diseases or illnesses that can mimic it such as a stroke. Even a seasoned neurologist can have difficulty in confirming a mild case of Parkinson's Disease because so many neurological conditions of other disorders imitate those of Parkinson's Disease.

The neurologists prescribed carbidopa/levodopa and Sinemet® for my father who eventually was treated with Requip. The most effective medication prescribed for treatment continues to be carbidopa/levodopa. When carbidopa is incorporated into levodopa, the chemical controls the conversion of levodopa into dopamine in the body's bloodstream by rerouting it to the brain and thereby reducing the needed dosage for treatment. Doctors must always weigh the potential benefits, risks, and other alternative medications for the unique treatment of Parkinson's Disease for each patient. Any delay in medical treatment always increases the fall risks for patients with Parkinson's Disease. Daddy suffered so much with nausea and an upset stomach while taking these medications.

To make matters worse, urologists diagnosed my dad with prostate cancer in 2001 after he underwent a painful biopsy. I have been told that prostate cancer is the "best cancer" a man can have, considering the fact that this type of cancer is slow growing and usually afflicts men over 80 years old. He also had a hydrocele which, according to *WebMD.com [March 26, 2017]*, is the collection of a watery fluid that surrounds one or both testicles. This condition has an ugly appearance and may cause discomfort, but my father was not in pain and in no danger. Doctors told me that draining the hydrocele was fruitless since it would return afterwards.

At this point in time, I had a consultation with Dr. Barry McKernan, a highly acclaimed surgeon specializing in laparoscopic surgery. Dr. McKernan has developed laparoscopic inguinal hernia repair, laparoscopic appendectomy, and other surgical procedures. For years I had been experiencing discomfort in and around the deep crevice [scar] in my side which was the surgical site for the emergency appendectomy performed in September 1975 that saved my life. This crevice in my right side is still there, undisturbed by other serious abdominal surgeries that have been performed afterwards. Dr. Knott referred me to Dr. McKernan, and the decision was made to perform surgery on May 15, 2003 to remove the adhesions and scar tissue that had formed and built up around this surgical site. On May 16 I began to suffer growing pain and discomfort in my abdomen, and I contacted Dr. McKernan's office on several occasions to let them know what I was experiencing. The doctors gave me stronger pain medication, but my condition was worsening by the hour. Finally, on May 17, after pacing the floor with severe abdominal pain most of the night, I spoke with Dr. Rick Finley, who had assisted in the previous operation, and he instructed me to go to Crawford Long Hospital where he would examine me. Ironically, this is the hospital where I was born and is a part of the prestigious and critically acclaimed Emory Health Care system.

I will never forget the telephone call I made to Joyce Crum at church on May 17 that I needed her to take me to Crawford Long Hospital as soon as possible. Joyce is a retired registered nurse in the United States Army, and she was helping me take care of my dad, transporting him to doctors' appointments. It was 1:00PM when Joyce came to the house to pick me and my father up and travel to the hospital in downtown Atlanta where we met with Dr. Finley. He ordered a CT scan to be performed to determine the possible cause of the abdominal pain and discomfort. The results of the CT scan: the surgery on May 15 had caused a tear in the intestinal wall which eventually created a blockage in the bowel, and a large abscess had formed in my rectum. Later I told a friend of mine about what had happened, and she said it sounded like a "botched" operation to her. The pain brought back memories of the excruciating agony and discomfort caused by the ruptured appendix in September 1975. I have to admit that I have no idea how I have endured and survived the excruciating pain and agony of concussions, collapsed lungs, and a ruptured appendix. But **Mark, Chapter 10, Verse 27 [New King James Version]**, says it all:

> "**²⁷ But Jesus looked at them and said, "With men *it is* impossible, but not with God; for with God all things are possible."**

At precisely 9:00PM I was wheeled into the operating room where I was placed on a cold and uncomfortable stainless steel operating table. Dr. Finley greeted me there, and he told me that he might have to perform a colostomy to save my life. A colostomy is a surgical procedure that brings one end of the large intestine out through the abdominal wall. During this procedure, one end of the colon is diverted through an incision in the abdominal wall to create a stoma. A stoma is the opening in the skin where a pouch for collecting feces is attached. People with colostomies, whether temporary or long-term, have pouches attached to their sides where feces collects and can be easily disposed of. Conditions that may warrant a permanent colostomy include a blockage in the colon or bowel. I literally pleaded with Dr. Finley not to remove my colon, if possible. I was terrified at the thought of having my active lifestyle altered in this way by being placed on disability or possibly not even surviving the operation altogether. Even in our darkest moments like these, I now recall God's promise that He made in **Joshua, Chapter 1, Verse 9 [New King James Version]**:

"⁹ Have I not commanded you? Be strong and of good courage; do not be afraid, nor be dismayed, for the LORD your God *is* with you wherever you go."

I recollect waking up right after the surgery, and I was wheeled down the hallways to the Intensive Care Unit [ICU] where I stayed for at least 2 days. When I have been in a hospital for surgery, I always think about the cool air coming from the air conditioning in the hallways blowing in my face when I am lying on the gurney. Later Daddy told me that Dr. Finley was supposed to call him after the surgery to give him an update. Daddy stayed up until 12:30AM, but Dr. Finley never called to inform him of the results of the operation. I remember lying on my back in a small room in the ICU. The moment I was clearly conscious, I felt my sides to see if I had a colostomy bag attached to my body. **When I discovered that there were no colostomy bags, my heart leaped for joy, and I thanked God for his grace and mercy in sparing my life yet once again for the 3ʳᵈ time.** At that point in time I was 52 years old which is the prime of life. Ron Lee-Own, my supervisor at the office at that time, came to see me in the ICU. I was deeply grateful for him to come to visit me in the hospital. I felt so isolated and alone in the bowels of the ICU, especially when an elderly patient passed away while I was there. His room was adjacent to mine. I can still hear the doctors and nurses scurrying about, and the cries for help from the family members of this dying man. This episode was not the last time that the Angel of Death would appear where I was.

The doctors put me on a morphine drip for the constant pain I had to endure because of the 2" deep, nearly foot long incision that had been carved into my abdomen. This incision is still a wicked looking scar on my stomach even after all these years have passed. I see it every day when I look in the mirror. Nurses had to change the bandages and dressing on the incision twice a day. I can still recall looking at the very deep and gruesome incision whenever the nurse changed the dressing in the hospital. I even had a nurse come to the house after I was released from the hospital to change the bandages. I also was not allowed to eat or drink fluids, and I was taking huge amounts of antibiotics to combat the infection deep inside my bowel. I had become susceptible to contracting sepsis which is a severe infection caused by bacteria and viruses in the blood or tissues. If this condition is left untreated, a localized infection [as in my case in the bowel] can spread to the bloodstream and cause widespread inflammation which can lead eventually to septic shock and even death. When I received my bill from the hospital for almost $40,000, medications amounted to $10,000 of the total bill. I had so many I-V bags that were draped on a pole with wheels on it. The I-V pole became my "buddy" as I was encouraged to move around, and I began to take laps around the hallway. Doctor's orders: 4 laps a day to regain my strength and speed up the healing process. It was all I could do to muster up enough energy and strength to navigate the hallway 2 times much less 4. When I was walking around, I was suffering with searing pain in my stomach. I was thankful for the morphine drip to control the pain and discomfort. I always felt like my guts were going to spill out all over the place at any time. The doctors had given me a tight elastic wrap to wear around my abdomen until after the end of the summer to help heal the incision. When friends visited me, they described me as being "white as a sheet". I was hospitalized for 2 weeks. My weight had plummeted to 147 pounds, the lowest it had been since I was in high school. I had to hold onto my pants because I had lost so much weight, and they were just too big for me to wear.

It took a long time for me to get stronger and gain the weight back. A doctor once told me that it can take more than a year to recover from major surgery. Ideally, I should have gone to the health club to exercise and regain my strength. But my father's health care took precedence over my own health and well-being from that point on until March 2006. That meant 7 days a week, 365 days a year non-stop. A important lesson I learned from my days at Innisbrook in enduring and surviving a mysterious illness is found in **Matthew, Chapter 6, Verses 25-34 [New King James Version]**, which gave me great comfort and I also saw on the wall of Dr. Hughes' office:

> "[25] **Therefore I say to you, do not worry about your life, what you will eat or what you will drink; nor about your body, what you will put on. Is not life more than food and the body more than clothing?** [26] **Look at the birds of the air, for they neither sow nor reap nor gather into barns; yet your heavenly Father feeds them. Are you not of more value than they?** [27] **Which of you by worrying can add one cubit to his stature?** [28] **So why**

do you worry about clothing? Consider the lilies of the field, how they grow: they neither toil nor spin; [29] and yet I say to you that even Solomon in all his glory was not arrayed like one of these. [30] Now if God so clothes the grass of the field, which today is, and tomorrow is thrown into the oven, *will He* not much more *clothe* you, O you of little faith? [31] Therefore do not worry, saying, 'What shall we eat?' or 'What shall we drink?' or 'What shall we wear?' [32] For after all these things the Gentiles seek. For your heavenly Father knows that you need all these things. [33] But <u>seek first the kingdom of God and His righteousness, and all these things shall be added to you.</u> [34] <u>Therefore do not worry about tomorrow, for tomorrow will worry about its own things. Sufficient for the day *is* its own trouble."</u>

Epicurus is quoted as saying "[i]t is not so much our friends' help that helps us, as the confidence of their help". My dad and I received so much assistance from our friends at the church as well as my coworkers at my office that it was overwhelming. I relied heavily on my friends to take my dad to doctor's appointments and to and from the hospital, buy groceries, and sometimes fix meals. It is a debt of gratitude that I can never repay for their kindness, generosity, and compassion at a time when I so desperately needed such. Members of McDonough First United Methodist Church who helped us include the following:

Karen DeVan
Betty and Jack Moore
Roxanne McManus, to name a few.

Members of Christ the King Lutheran Church in Peachtree Corners, Georgia that helped my dad and me are the following:

Joyce and Ray Crum
Ruth and Don Harrivel
Bill Jensen

Pat and Bob McNally
Susie and Glenn McGuffin
Les Sheridan
Pastor Landa Larson
Jennifer Fischer
John Rhodes
Lynn Yearous
Jan Arnson
Sondra Einig

My co-workers at my office were so supportive and generous during our time of need and never-ending crisis:

Eve Schultz
Ron Lee-Own
Redding Davis
Joe Reach
Ken Baker
Sam Blackburn
Fran Osteen
Steve Bayne
Fran Nowak
Jerold Davis
Tom Presley
Cheryl McGriff, and so many others.

They were always there when we were so disheartened and overwhelmed. Without them and Marilyn and Mandy, I would not have survived. Dwight L. Moody once said that "**[f]aith makes all things possible.....love makes all things easy.**"

I considered it such a great honor and privilege to have the responsibility for taking care of my dad. But I was so overcome by the daunting task of taking care of him and my own health problems, I was afraid of losing my job with the State of Florida. All of my vacation and sick leave had been consumed during the recovery from the 2 abdominal surgeries in May 2003. I finally returned to work on July 14, 2003 on a part-time basis per doctor's orders because I did not want to overdo it due to my still weakened physical condition, and I was given a huge unfinished audit assignment to work on upon my return. What is so unbelievable is I actually began to jog again in September 2003 after 15 years of not being able to run or jog. I started jogging slowly and even walking uphill with a gallon bottle of water in my arms to strengthen my lower back and stomach muscles which had been devastated by the 2 abdominal surgeries.

During the week of Thanksgiving in 2003, Daddy fell during the night and broke his left arm right at the top of his shoulder. This injury would change our lives from that point on. The doctors could do nothing but place his left arm in a sling for 6 weeks. For the first time I had to have assistance at the house because there was no way I could lift my father out of bed or help him move around the house during the day when I was at work. Mandy advised me to have *Home Instead Senior Care* come to take care of my dad and to eventually place him in a nearby assisted living facility. Because the assisted living facilities require a 2-day TB test for a new patient and the upcoming holiday weekend was upon us, we were unable to get Daddy into the facility until the following week. *Home Instead Senior Care*, a non-medical home care and elderly companionship service provider, charged us a total of $2,600 for one week of care which, believe or not, is not covered by Medicare. My dad stayed at the assisted living facility for 1 year until December 2004. Again the cost of assisted living is not covered by Medicare. The problems we encountered while my father was there were the difficulty of finding staff to help you on the weekends, slow response to requests for assistance from the staff, a frigid temperature in the room and the inability to get the facility to adjust the thermostat, and a leak in the roof above my dad's room so bad we had to put a bucket under it to catch the rainwater. Another unsettling concern was the constant traffic of other patients coming into my father's room during the night uninvited.

When we moved my father into the assisted living facility in Roswell, my Stephen minister helped us bring some furniture from our house on his trailer for my dad's room that he would have to share soon with another gentleman. For some inexplicable reason, he left the TV set on the floor instead of placing it on top of the dresser like I asked him to. I could not find anyone in the building to pick up the TV set off the floor. Even though I had just had major abdominal surgeries 6 months ago, I believed I could still pick up the TV set without hurting myself. But I was dead wrong. I would later be diagnosed with an umbilical cord hernia which I suffered after lifting the TV set. To this day I still cannot understand why he had plopped the TV set on the floor and then left without saying a word. Unbelievable and irresponsible behavior on his part.

On April 14, 2005, Dr. Finley performed the laparoscopic surgery to repair the umbilical hernia. A laparoscope is a thin, lighted tube that enables the surgeon to see inside the abdomen. According to *MedLine Plus Medical Encyclopedia [March 26, 2017]*, an umbilical hernia is a pouch that has been made from the inner lining of the stomach. This pouch eventually pushes through a hole that has emerged in the wall of the stomach at the navel. Umbilical hernias tend to grow in size over time and become painful so surgery becomes necessary to repair the hole or weak spot caused by the hernia. Successful surgery restores stability to the weakened abdominal wall tissue and repairs any holes.

Dr. Finley had to lay a large piece of mesh over the weakened area that was anchored by hooks and strong stitches to make it stronger. I had successful outpatient hernia repair surgery and was allowed to go home even though Dr. Finley had recommended and insisted I stay overnight because of my past medical history. I can still remember the excruciating and piercing pain in my stomach whenever I tried to get up out of a chair or even to bend over. Just unbelievable searing pain! It would take a long time for me to recover from the hernia surgery. For what seemed like an eternity I could not stand up straight when I was walking because of the lingering pain from the surgery. Please refer to *MedLine Plus Medical Encyclopedia* for more detailed information about umbilical hernias.

Almost 3 weeks after this serious surgery, my father complained of chest discomfort. He had not complained before about the heaviness in his chest. Before this episode, my dad had been hospitalized for the first time with a blood clot in his left thigh which was discovered by an ultrasound examination in a doctor's office. The doctors prescribed Warfarin or Coumadin for Daddy which is an anticoagulant normally used in the prevention of blood clots forming in the blood vessels and their potential movement to somewhere else in the body. The use of Warfarin or Coumadin has to be monitored regularly by blood testing to ensure an adequate yet safe dose is being taken.

It was 4:00 on a Saturday afternoon, and I was beside myself as to what to do for him. Daddy suggested contacting his Stephen minister Glenn McGuffin to see if he could take us to the emergency room at the hospital on such a short notice. Glenn was so gracious to come to our house and take us to North Fulton Regional Hospital in Roswell. He and his wife Susie are still close friends, and they were there at my dad's bedside when he passed away. Doctors at the hospital diagnosed that my dad had pericarditis or the inflammation of the pericardium. According to *WebMD.com* [March 26, 2017], this inflammation causes a buildup of an abnormal amount of fluid between the heart and the pericardium which is a tough, layered sac surrounding the heart. This condition impairs heart function because the heart cannot slide easily within the pericardium when it is beating.

After undergoing surgery to remove 100 cc of fluid around his heart, the doctors ultimately diagnosed my father with congestive heart failure and prescribed Digoxin. Mandy was surprised that he had survived the surgery, but Dr. Moribaldi, the chiropractor whose steadfast and fervent care kept him going, would later say that my dad had such a strong "life force". The *Mayo Clinic* [March 27, 2017] describes the use of Digoxin for treatment of congestive heart failure by improving the strength and performance of the heart or to control the efficiency of the heartbeat, resulting in better circulation.

Tragically, adding to my dad's woes, he was exposed to and contracted C. *diff* in the hospital. According to *WebMD.com* [March 27, 2017], Clostridium difficile (C. difficile, or C. diff) is a relatively rare bacteria that exists among 1,000 other species of other microorganisms in the stomach and intestines. In a healthy digestive tract, these microorganisms are basically harmless and sometimes work together. However, if an organism ever interferes with the interaction of these organisms in the stomach, harmless bacteria can make a person ill if they spiral out of control. Some of these bacteria can no longer keep in check the C-diff bacteria which is one of the leading causes of infectious diarrhea. This C-diff infection can be mild in duration with watery diarrhea or life-threatening as it releases poisons to destroy the lining of the intestines. C. diff is most likely to affect patients in hospitals or long-term care facilities where Daddy had been cared for.

My father suffered horribly with C. diff. He had "accidents" because at times he could not control his bowel movements. He had to wear Depend diapers which were so embarrassing to him. Daddy would urinate in his Depends to avoid having to get up to go to the bathroom. I finally got a portable toilet to make it so much easier for him to go to the bathroom. In the other extreme, medications made him constipated. One day I had to help him to go to the bathroom by digital removal of his bowel movements. He suffered so much with "hard stools".

His quality of life was slowly but surely slipping away from him. One day Mandy reminded me that my father had a terminal illness in Parkinson's Disease which hit me like "a load of bricks". Thank God for the compassionate and knowledgeable caregivers like Janice Cox as well as Ann and Jane who were assigned to us by At Home Personal Care through Mandy Merkel to give him comfort and companionship. They helped me during the day by taking care of my dad when I was at work. **Mother Teresa, who shares the same birthday as mine [August 26], once said that "[p]eace begins with a smile".** Both ladies were from Kenya, and they were always smiling, like angels in disguise. Of course, I was always there in the evenings to be with my father. It was 7 days a week, 24 hours a day with no vacations or time off for good behavior. I gave Daddy a bath, usually on Saturdays, and trimmed his toenails to the best of my ability. I helped him put on his shoes because bending over was so difficult for him. But it was a privilege and an honor for me to take care of my father. My main objective was to keep him out of a nursing home and to stay in our home until the end finally came. I did not want my father to suffer the same fate my mother did, dying in a nursing home among strangers. Mission accomplished.

I purchased a record player for Daddy that could play 78's containing Big Band music, George Gershwin, Ernie Ford, Perry Como, Andy Williams, and the huge collection of classical music composed by Bach, Beethoven, Brahms, Chopin, Mozart, Rachmaninoff, Tchaikovsky, and Wagner. I also bought a CD player which played the CDs containing the Big Band sound of Glenn Miller, Benny Goodman, Harry James, Tommy Dorsey, Lionel Hampton, Vaughn Monroe, and Artie Shaw. One of his favorite movies was *The Glenn Miller Story* [1954] starring James Stewart and June Allyson. My dad got such great enjoyment from listening to music. Lawrence Welk and the *Bee Gees* were also his favorites. We had the great pleasure twice to watch the live concert performed by the *Bee Gees* in 1997. I still remember filling the air of our house with Christmas music in 2005, the last Christmas of Daddy's life.

My father loved the litany and liturgy of the Lutheran church because we sang the canticles, anthems, and the sacraments similar to those of the Catholic Church. With his Lutheran upbringing in mind, I felt that we should join a Lutheran church in the local area despite the fact that we had been going to Methodist churches for quite some time. I thank God we joined Christ the King Lutheran Church in Norcross shortly after our move from Stockbridge to Roswell in late December 2001. After all these years, I owed it to my father to join a Lutheran church for his sake. Pastor Landa, Joyce Crum, and Pat McNally would come from the church frequently to visit with Daddy to lift up his spirits.

Dr. Mike Moribaldi was a chiropractor and a fellow Mason like us. If my memory serves me correctly, Mike served the Masonic Lodge as the Worshipful Master. Whenever we went to see Dr. Mike on Saturdays, afterwards we headed for Wendy's or Arby's. The common refrain from my dad was "a burger and a shake" for lunch on our Saturday excursions. Dr. Mike made a few house calls to take care of Daddy whenever possible. Craig Storlie, a "jack of all trades" in home improvements and repairing anything mechanical, was there at the house to replace the tile in the bath tubs in both bathrooms. He also installed grab bars in each bath tub to help prevent falls while taking a bath. What was so miraculous to me was how Craig built wooden ramps in just over an hour to allow easy access for my dad's wheelchair to go up and over the front steps and the steps in the foyer. It made everything so much easier to cope with my father's lack of mobility and an increased use of the wheelchair. Just amazing! Jill Knueppel, Craig's wife and a neuromuscular massage therapist, came to the house to work on both Daddy and myself. Believe or not, Craig and Jill are both ordained Lutheran ministers.

Mischief, our beloved Schnauzer, was my constant, faithful companion whenever Daddy was in the hospital during 2005 and 2006. She was always there to give me comfort at home and would stay in the car and snooze when I was in the hospital room for a visit. Mischief had visited him in the assisted living facility where she was allowed to come into his room and also pay a visit with the other residents. I would go out to the parking lot and take Mischief for a long walk. In December 1999 she was struck down by a mysterious illness caused by elevated liver enzymes. Daddy and I had rescued Mischief from the Henry County dog pound where she had been exposed to polluted water, contaminated food, and disease. This hostile environment had obviously affected her physical health and well-being. The vet at the hospital said that she would not make it through the weekend before Christmas. We thought we had lost Mischief, but she somehow survived to take care of both of us. It was a great Christmas gift to see her tail wagging when we walked into the back of the hospital. The vet replied she was going to pull through after all. A great sadness for me was losing our beloved dog Mischief on February 16, 2006. I had noticed earlier that she had swollen glands when I felt around her neck area. She would be eventually diagnosed with lymphoma by Dr. Joe Gaston after receiving the lab work results, and he gave her maybe 12 months at the most to live. Mischief choked to death right at my feet in front of the fireplace. I felt so helpless that there was totally nothing I could do to save her that morning. I still cannot believe the sadness and grief caused by the loss of such a faithful friend. Even Ann was moved to tears as she placed Mischief in my car for the final trip to the vet for cremation.

On January 27, 2006 I came down with a highly contagious virus that was going around the office at the time. Thank God, up to that point, after over 4 years had passed, I had miraculously been able to stay healthy and strong since 2003. But it was a serious illness that eventually turned into double pneumonia. I was so sick with a high fever and a terrible cough that I missed considerable time from work. Tragically my father caught this virus from being around me, and he, too, came down with pneumonia. He had to be hospitalized for a few days, and I could sense that he was beginning to give up the fight to go on. Nevertheless, Daddy kept his uncontainable sense of humor, and when a nurse came into my dad's hospital room and asked him if he needed anything, his simple response was "a rich widow".

I remember that the weather was so cold and damp most of February 2006. One Sunday morning I was watching Jentezen Franklin on Trinity Broadcasting Network. Our circumstances were so dire and discouraging that I felt so overwhelmed and depressed. My father's hospital bills were $250,000, and we eventually spent over $80,000 out of pocket for his health care. We were quite simply running out of money, our life savings. In his sermon Franklin emphasized that we should always praise the Lord at all times, good or bad. God expects us to do so no matter how dire and overwhelming our circumstances seem to be. In **Psalm 34**, **Verse 1** [**New**

King James Version], it says that **"I will bless the Lord at all times no matter what my circumstances; His praise shall continually be in my mouth."** Daddy asked me one day: "Who is going to take care of you, David, after I'm gone?" All I could say in reply is God will take good care of me. He was always so concerned about my health and well-being, but so is God. Mandy Merkel recommended that my dad be placed in hospice care on February 20, 2006. It was the beginning of the end. Unfortunately, for my father, his fate was already sealed, and it was too late to save him. He not only was battling Parkinson's Disease but also congestive heart failure, prostate cancer, Restless Legs Syndrome, and acid reflux.

In late February the NCAA basketball season was gearing up for the finale that has been hailed for decades as *March Madness*. Every year Daddy and I always looked forward to following the tournament since the 1960's when the UCLA Bruins were so dominant under fabled coach John Wooden. We are rabid Duke fans, and the ACC tournament was right around the corner. But Florida was the eventual champion in 2006. Joyce Crum reminded me to **cherish the moments that you have with your loved ones**. My dad and I always enjoyed watching sporting events together, whether it be the NFL, NBA, or college level. He would play catch with a baseball or shoot baskets with me when I was growing up. We jogged together for a long time and enjoyed sailing for 30 years. We built the basketball backboard in the backyard over the carport that we also built ourselves. We laid concrete blocks to reinforce the driveway in the back and made concrete grills. I learned simple carpentry skills just being around my dad which I still use to this day. I really miss his fatherly wisdom and guidance which cannot be duplicated. He would say "calm seas a Captain does not make". Each day he reminded me: "Who are you going to serve today, David?" As Joshua said, "as for me and my house, I will serve the Lord".

I started to work at home more often. I became somewhat paranoid whenever I heard the telephone ring at the office, thinking that something was wrong with my father and I would have to drop everything I was doing and return home to face yet another crisis. It was March 9, 2006, exactly 3 weeks after Mischief had passed away. Jennifer Fischer, a member of Christ the King and a hospice nurse, visited with my dad and me that fateful day. After Jennifer saw him, she told us that my dad was in the stage of slowly dying. My audit work was such a blessing because it kept my mind, what was left of it, on something else besides our dire circumstances.

About 8:30PM Daddy began to have great difficulty breathing after Ann had fed him that evening. He asked for blueberry jam, and Ann gave my dad some to eat. I was in a state of denial that the end of my father's life was near. We contacted Pastor Landa who came and tried her best to comfort me. Jennifer Fischer and Glenn and Susie McGuffin also joined us there, and I was holding my father's hand when he breathed his last at 11:55PM. Ann had left for the evening, and she was so despondent that she had not been there for us at the end. I remember now that Mother had passed away at almost exactly the same time around midnight on December 4, 1993.

On November 15, 2015 Pastor John Weber gave a sermon about the end of time really being just the beginning of eternal life. *The End* it was called. **T H E stands for Trust, Hope, and Empowerment. E N D stands for Every New Day**. But I will never forget the ominous silence that consumed the house the next day, March 10. I had gone to bed around 2:00AM, in shock from what had transpired at midnight. Glenn was so kind to stay with me that sad night. I took something to help me get whatever sleep I could get. I had been spending so much time in the company of death. A portion of the epitaph written for my great friend Kaye Neuman, who lived outside Clearwater, Florida and had passed away earlier, contains a fitting tribute to my father:

> **"....In life we loved you dearly,**
> **In death we do the same,**
> **It broke our hearts to lose you,**
> **....For part of us went with you,**
> **....Our family chain is broken,**
> **And nothing seems the same,**
> **But as God calls us one by one,**
> **The chain will link again."**

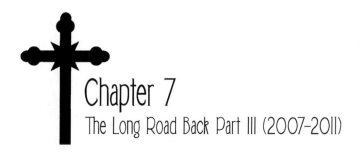

Chapter 7
The Long Road Back Part III (2007-2011)

Taking care of my dad had taken such a tremendous toll on my health not only physically but also spiritually and emotionally. I was so totally drained after losing my 2 best friends exactly 3 weeks apart. I had literally sacrificed my own health to take care of both Daddy and Mischief. During this time it was impossible for me to exercise properly or work out like I had done in the past. But I did begin to jog in September 2003 and have never stopped. Sometimes I had to eat on the run and at different hours of the day. I am thankful that my audit work had kept my mind occupied, but **what was so amazing to me was that I did not lose my job with the State of Florida**. In fact, I had excelled in my audit work despite the distractions, pressures, stress, and the great sadness of taking care of my dad every single day for over 4 years. I was working on 10 huge audit assignments that would come to a successful conclusion in 2007. I guess daily life is a constant struggle to adapt to survive and prosper by facing life's challenges through our faith in God and our Lord Jesus Christ. We all have to deal with loss at some time during our lives. I now came to the realization that I had no family living in the state of Georgia. The closest family that I had lived in and around the Charlotte, North Carolina area. Pastor Dave Koppel, the senior pastor at Christ the King at that time, encouraged me by saying that the church would now be my new family. That statement became my motto from that point on.

Misty, the miniature Schnauzer, came into my life on April 2, 2006, *the same exact same day Mischief's dog tag expired*. I had found this wonderful little dog with a big heart on *PetFinder.com*. As I said before, Jessica and Ron Christian, a young couple with 4 small children, who lived in Johnson City, Tennessee, could no longer take care of this sweet mild-mannered 3-year old dog. Misty was a gift from Daddy for taking care of him, Mandy said. My father's birthday is April 4 which he just missed by a month. Even though Misty felt right at home from the outset, she looked up at me the day I brought her home and asked me with her facial expression if this is her new home and if I was going to take care of her. I never felt so alone in a big house. Misty was a calm, affectionate dog who loved everybody. She never met a stranger and became my constant companion on trips to see family and go to Stone Mountain Park, Lake Lanier Islands, the Chattahoochee River trails, and Kennesaw Mountain National Battlefield for fun and relaxation. I also resumed jogging and working out regularly at the local YMCA in October 2006. I tried to get back into the swing of things, some kind of normalcy, regain some form of sanity.

However, during the remainder of 2006 and well into 2007, I struggled with colon problems, loose bowel movements, and regular diarrhea. Much to my dismay and disgust, Atlanta Gastroenterology misdiagnosed my health problems and eventually prescribed Questran for me. *Wikipedia, the Free Encyclopedia [March 27, 2017]* describes Questran as a medication commonly used to treat diarrhea resulting from the malabsorption of bile acid. It is still almost inconceivable for me to fathom why Atlanta Gastroenterology had prescribed Questran in powder form inside 4-g packets for the treatment of a dysfunctional gallbladder which was causing my diarrhea and colon discomfort. In January 2008 I began to have more pain and discomfort on the right side of my abdomen. Dr. David Clifford, my primary care physician at the time, examined me and ordered an ultrasound of my abdomen. The test results indicated the presence of gallstones, which are solidified particles of substances in the bile, and I was referred immediately to Dr. Matthew J. Novak, a specialist in general surgery. Gallstones can be as tiny as a grain of sand or the size of a golf ball.

In its Internet website *LiveScience.com [March 27, 2017]* provides information about the gallbladder which produces, stores, and transports bile, a yellowish-brown fluid that is generated from the liver for use in tearing up fatty substances for digestion in the small intestine. According to Great Britain's *National Health Service*, a patient can survive without the gallbladder because the bile can flow into the small intestine from other sources.

According to the *National Institutes of Health's* Internet website *[March 27, 2017]*, a gallbladder attack is characterized by sudden pain and discomfort usually caused by the blockage of the bile ducts by gallstones. A gallbladder attack can continue for several hours or for shorter periods of time. The *University of California-San Francisco Department of Surgery* emphasizes that the symptoms of a gallbladder attack mimic those of a heart attack and other medical conditions. The following symptoms of a gallbladder attack have been compiled by the *University of Maryland Medical Center*:

- Nausea or vomiting, including severe heartburn which I experienced after eating a meal
- Loss of appetite
- Pain and discomfort primarily in the upper right side of the abdomen.

Under *LiveScience.com [March 27, 2017]*, the *Mayo Clinic* states that doctors often recommend surgical removal of the gallbladder when the presence of gallstones is found. On February 6, 2008, Dr. Novak finally performed laparoscopic surgery, the least invasive surgical procedure, to remove my gallbladder. I had suffered with problems with digestion and loose bowel for at least 10 years. I had to sacrifice my health during that time in order to take care of my dad and continue to work. It took 2 years for me to fully recover from the surgery as I agonized with frequent trips to the bathroom and "accidents" where I could not make it to the restroom and ruined my clothing. But these lingering symptoms eventually dissipated.

A year later during 2009 I began to face the first of 2 seemingly insurmountable challenges simultaneously. I had been suffering with bouts of prostatitis and was being treated with antibiotics by Dr. Lewis Kriteman, a urologist in Roswell, who also had taken care of my father. Daddy called the urologist "the rear admiral" for obvious reasons when the doctor performed a digital rectal exam of the prostate. Dr. Kriteman had been watching my prostate specific androgen (PSA) carefully ever since my dad had been diagnosed with prostate cancer in 2002. In its Internet website *Cancer Treatment Centers of America [March 27, 2017]* has made the observation that the symptoms of prostate cancer, which can differ for each man, are not even noticeable in the early stages of the disease. Dr. Kriteman told me that the normal range of the PSA for a man at the age of 55 and over is 3.0 through 4.5. Digital rectal exams (DRE) and PSA are recommended for routine screenings, especially as declared by the

American Cancer Society who recommends men to be tested for prostate cancer, beginning at the age of 50. When my PSA had steeped to 5.7, Dr. Kriteman decided that I should undergo a biopsy, a medical procedure my dad had undergone and had had a painful reaction to it. Per articles found in *eMedicine Health.com [March 27, 2017]*, a biopsy, which removes samples of tissue in the prostate, is usually performed as an outpatient procedure whenever the doctor's findings uncovered by the physical exam, DRE, and PSA level or velocity indicate the presence of cancer. A pathologist, who specializes in diagnosing diseases, examines the sample of tumor tissue through a microscope to verify the presence of prostate cancer and makes an important assessment or grade called the Gleason score from the specimens taken. This indicator is so critical because the score is a measurement of the potential growth of the cancer cells and dictates what the possible treatment plan will be. The Gleason score can even reveal the chances of a cure after treatment. Whenever the Gleason score is 6 or lower, the prostate cancer is not aggressive and thus has a low grade rating. Any Gleason score that ranges from 8 to 10 is considered to be more aggressive cancer and, therefore, has a high grade rating. Unfortunately my Gleason score was 7 which is assessed somewhere between 8 and 10. The great news for most men like myself is prostate cancer generally responds well to treatments which vary according to the severity of the disease defined by stage of the tumor, Gleason score, and PSA level. Listed below are various options to treat localized prostate cancer:

- Active surveillance
- Radical prostatectomy
- Radiation therapy
- Cryotherapy and High-Intensity Focused Ultrasound

Other treatments available to attack advanced prostate cancer include hormonal therapy and chemotherapy.

It is very important for all the health care professionals involved, including the urologist and the cancer specialist or oncologist, to collaborate in order to fashion and design a unique treatment plan for each man based upon his expectations, explicit necessities, and concerns or uncertainty surrounding the success of the different options available.

My battle against prostate cancer began upon the results of the biopsy being revealed to me on May 18, 2010. I knew that I had cancer after undergoing the biopsy which had caused me so much pain and discomfort not only in the area of the prostate but also in my lower back and spine. I suffered with this pain for 2 days after the biopsy was performed. The biopsy results indicated 5 out of 12 samples of tissue taken from the prostate were malignant. It was determined that 2 out of the 5 malignant tissue samples were **aggressive cancer**. The urologist discussed different options for treatment of the prostate cancer, and it was decided that I would undergo 25 radiation treatments and 2 seed implant surgeries as soon as possible. However, my radiation treatments would be delayed until other tests and examinations were performed.

My agonizing odyssey began shortly thereafter in June 2010 with a bone scan, CT scans, PET scan, and numerous lab and blood work performed to verify if the cancer had possibly spread (metastasized) to other organs and other parts of my body. The test results showed the presence of bilateral inguinal hernias, but no evidence of other cancer was found. **What is so astonishing to me is that on June 30, 2009 Dr. Bonnie Hayes, a chiropractor and kinesiologist, had examined me and found problems with my left lung that should be properly diagnosed and treated by specialists. However, Dr. Hayes did not elaborate as to what the nature of the lung problem was.**

On June 30, 2010 Dr. Dan Callahan, a pulmonary specialist, ordered a bronchoscopy to be performed as an outpatient procedure. In its Internet website the *National Heart, Lung, and Blood Institute [March 27, 2017]* discusses in detail the nature and purpose of a bronchoscopy which is a medical procedure performed basically to determine the cause of a problem in the lungs by examining the airways carrying air from the trachea to the lungs. The pulmonary specialist uses the bronchoscope, a slender and elastic or a rigid tube, to enter into the airways of the lungs through the nose for the purpose of detecting and identifying any tumors, possible infection, excessive layers of mucus, bleeding, or blockage in the airways. The bronchoscope has a light and small camera that allows the doctor to see the windpipe and airways and the opportunity to take pictures as well as tissue or mucus samples from the lungs for testing in a laboratory. This medical procedure, which can be done in a hospital operating room using general anesthesia, is occasionally performed to treat the lung problems. **Whether it is prophetic or not, almost exactly a year later after being examined by Dr. Hayes, the blood and lab work, including cultures taken from lung tissues during the bronchoscopy, was completed on July 13, 2010. Thanks be to God that all test results and cultures were negative; however, 1 culture unfortunately contained the *Mycobacterium avium-intracellulare* infection (MAI), also known as MAC (Mycobacterium Avium Complex) which was going to plague my life for over 2 years**.

In its Internet website *MedScape.com* [March 28, 2017] describes *M avium complex* (MAC) as a fungal infection that causes disease in humans through the inhalation of airborne organisms created in an environment such as water, soil, dust, and various animals. It has been determined that I suffer with **chronic bronchiectasis** which falls into 1 of 2 patterns of MAC disease in patients like myself with underlying lung disease. Bronchiectasis is the bronchial condition which causes unnatural enlargement of the bronchial tubes with small, ill-defined nodules. This particular lung disease appears to be a common denominator associated with MAC infection. It is still unclear whether or not bronchiectasis leads to or results from the MAC infection. Coughing is the most common symptom of this disease which I myself can attest to.

The recommended treatment for patients with MAC infection includes daily ethambutol, rifampicin or rifabutin, and clarithromycin or azithromycin. The length of medical treatment with antibiotics should be at least 12 months. Surgery is also an option which includes lung resection for patients where medications have failed. I was treated with antibiotics by Dr. Michael Dailey, a board-certified infectious disease specialist, for 24 long months—ethambutol, rifampicin, and azithromycin. My stomach just could not tolerate taking rifampicin on an empty stomach in the morning because I became so nauseated and sick to my stomach when I took the medication. MAC can cause fever and diarrhea as well as loss of appetite, fatigue, and weight loss, and can spread to the bone marrow where anemia and low white blood cell count can develop.

From May 18, 2010 I lived in fear and apprehension that I might lose my life to cancer and/or lung disease. Fortunately, I realized that prostate cancer is slow-growing and can be successfully treated if detected in time. From the outset I literally felt the prayers of so many friends and family, especially the church, that I never felt alone. **Please keep in mind that I was not only battling prostate cancer but at the same time I was also fighting a serious lung infection**. My first lung infection occurred in September 1967 and was diagnosed by Dr. Rodriguez at Piedmont Hospital. This was the first of several "lung infections" that I have suffered during my lifetime.

Christopher Reeve said it best. "A hero is an ordinary individual who finds the strength to persevere and endure in spite of overwhelming obstacles." I underwent a total of 25 radiation treatments which finally began on August 3, 2010. Each treatment averaged 20 minutes in duration and occurred each weekday until September 9, 2010. I lay totally motionless on a cold stainless steel table for each treatment. In addition, on August 20 and August 27, 2010, I underwent back to back **High Dosage Radiation [HDR] therapy** which is also called **seed implant surgery**. The day of the surgery I arrived at North Fulton Regional Hospital at 6:00 in the morning for the first phase of the HDR therapy. Don Harrivel, a member of Christ the King, was kind enough to take me to the hospital for both surgeries. There at the hospital Dr. Kriteman gave me a painful injection in my lower back that paralyzed me from the waist down. For the second phase I was then taken by ambulance to the nearby office of Dr. Craig Wilkinson, the oncologist, where I was placed in the HDR Therapy Room which had no windows and was dark. Approximately 17 catheters were inserted inside my prostate during both surgical procedures.

To say the least, the 2nd and last HDR therapy scared me spitless. The HDR therapy room was so small that I became claustrophobic and terrified. Each seed implant surgery took an excruciating 20 to 30 minutes. Maybe I inherited my claustrophobia from my grandfather who was a coal miner and worked for decades in close quarters within the confines of the mine shaft. Dee Donnelly, a retired ordained minister and member of Christ the King, contacted me, and we discussed the aspects and trauma of undergoing radiation treatments and the seed implant surgery. I broke down and sobbed about the fears I had of being in the HDR therapy room. Her husband Jim came the day before the 2nd HDR therapy which happened to be August 26, my 60th birthday. Jim stayed with me all afternoon and into the evening to give me comfort and reassurance that I would survive the surgical procedure with "flying colors". What a way to celebrate a milestone birthday. This last HDR therapy introduced me to the drug Zanax which Dr. Wilkinson prescribed just for the surgery. According to *WebMD.com [March 28, 2017]*, Zanax is a medication which is used to treat anxiety and panic disorders by producing a calming effect.

I suffered so much not only physically but also mentally and emotionally. The radiation treatments did not hurt or cause me any discomfort. But the unknown outcome of the radiation treatments and the length of time required for taking powerful antibiotics for the lung infection weighed heavily on my mind. Weight loss was dramatic during the radiation treatments which worried me even more. My weight plummeted down below 160 pounds for the 1st time since June 2003. I also experienced significant changes in my bowel movements. On a few occasions after I parked my car across the street, the moment I walked over to the building where I was undergoing the radiation treatments I had to rush to the restroom. I had this happen on several other occasions following the radiation treatments. I suffered with great fatigue for a long time which was directly caused by the radiation. To this day I still fight fatigue of some degree each day.

During these radiation treatments, members of Christ the King Lutheran Church came over to our house to do yard work such as mowing the lawn, trimming the shrubbery, spreading gravel for the path in the back yard around the deck, and, more significantly, repainting the interior of the house to get it ready for sale later in 2012. In January 2010 I had applied for refinancing and restructuring of the mortgages encumbering the house, and to my great dismay I could not consolidate the debt on the house because the bank appraisal of the property was lower than expected. It was a crushing blow, considering my total health care costs for 2010 were a staggering $230,000. Without the insurance coverage with Blue Cross/Blue Shield and AFLAC, I would have been wiped out financially. I still consider the unexpected money I received from AFLAC in the amount of approximately $14,000 a bona fide miracle. God indeed provides for us.

Upon my return to the office in late October 2010, I was required to prepare for overnight travel for audit assignments. Because I was in such a weak physical condition, I had hoped for a gradual return to the office and resumption of working on audit assignments and eventually performing audit field work. I felt like I was "under the microscope" by top management to see if I could still "cut the mustard" by sending me out in the field as soon as possible. I already had 2 overnight audit assignments waiting for me when I arrived back in the office. The audit field work would be performed in the Muscle Shoals, Alabama area which was 300 miles away from our house in Roswell. I became fearful of a relapse because of the great stress of being on the road again and "living out of a suitcase" in a hotel as well as working with taxpayer personnel who did not want me there in the first place. **Please remember that I was going to be under the continuing care of Dr. Kriteman and Dr. Wilkinson for the long-term recovery from prostate cancer as well as following the heavy antibiotic protocol for treatment of a serious lung infection <u>until August 2012</u> under the continuing care of Dr. Callahan and Dr. Dailey.**

On the road the hotel room became a "chamber of horrors" for me for the first time because of the claustrophobic surroundings in the room. I had been traumatized by my unsettling experiences inside the HDR therapy room. I found it extremely difficult just to relax so that I could go to sleep at night. Compounding the problem was my continuing battle with fatigue. I had been taking Restoril or Temazepam since 1989 as a sleep aid prescribed by Dr. Knott. *Drugs.com [March 27, 2017]* states that Restoril relieves insomnia symptoms which basically involve trouble falling or staying asleep. Sometimes I would walk during the night in the hallways outside the hotel room, trying to calm myself down so that I could go back to bed to get a good night's sleep. I knew that the lack of sleep and rest could adversely affect my audit performance.

I told doctors that I was beginning to have self-doubt and anxiety about my future and physical well-being. The doctor prescribed Lexapro which *WebMD.com [March 27, 2017]* describes as a medication which treats both depression and anxiety and also energizes the patient as well as helps restore the feelings of well-being. The use of Lexapro did not seem to relieve my feelings of hopelessness and nervousness. Anxiety began to dominate my thinking, even when I was away from the "pressure cooker" office environment. Doctors then prescribed Zanax for me after I let them know about the ineffectiveness of Lexapro in my treatment of anxiety and nervousness which seemed to be spiraling out of control.

Buddha once observed that "**[y]ou, yourself, as much as anybody in the entire universe, deserve your love and affection.**" During the early part of 2011, I earnestly began to dream about and visualize retirement in the not too distant future. Retirement was a milestone I thought I would never achieve in my wildest dreams because of the serious health problems I had faced and overcome. In August 2012 I would turn 62, and I later discovered that I could retire at that age with full pension benefits from the State of Florida. I could also begin drawing Social Security benefits early. Thomas Alva Edison said that **"[m]any of life's failures are people who did not realize how close they were to success when they gave up"**. But Mr. Edison did not consider the effects of depression and feelings of despair on the mind and the will to overcome and succeed in the midst of dire and seemingly hopeless circumstances.

My first bout of depression and anxiety came in 1970 when I was a sophomore attending Georgia State University. After the disappointing experience I had had with dormitory life at Catawba College, I lived at home with my parents during the entire time I attended Georgia State. From January 1969 until the end of Spring Quarter of 1970 I was constantly going to college and studying so hard that I had no social life whatsoever. The only time off I had away from going to school was between quarters. I was majoring in accounting and eventually mathematics, but I was buried in taking meaningless courses in English literature, chemistry, psychology, and sociology which have absolutely nothing to do with business and accounting. I literally became "burnt out" with school and began to suffer through depression, increasing self-doubt, low self-esteem, and the fear of failure which I had never experienced before. I had always "raised the bar high" when it came to maintaining straight A's in my school work and studies. Those had been my standards of excellence in school no matter what. But I was now beginning to take accounting and other business courses that were going to be a true challenge for me. My self-confidence was being severely tested. Since high school my entire life had revolved around getting my college degree. I finally received psychological counseling for the first time at Georgia State. Nevertheless, I "limped" the rest of my college days as I struggled to get through each course and finally get my BBA degree in June 1973. I just hated going to school. I was burnt out with it.

Over 40 years later, in June 2011, I was feeling more and more overwhelmed by my circumstances. It would take a long time for me to recover from the prostate cancer treatments so that I could even resume a normal routine, much less working as hard as I could in my audit work. Earlier in October 2010 I had gone to Atlanta Gastroenterology where the doctors found acute inflammation in my rectum by using a sigmoidoscope. The inflammation had been caused by the radiation treatments and the seed implant surgeries for aggressive prostate cancer. I eventually received treatment from Dr. Wilkinson, in the form of *Proctofoam HC* which I sprayed inside my rectum 3 times a day. In its Internet website *Drugs.com* [*March 28, 2017*], it is explained that the medication *Proctofoam* contains Hydrocortisone, a steroid, and a topical compound that treat and reduce pain, inflammation, itching, redness, and swelling of the skin caused by a number of conditions, including **the rectal area.**

Life sometimes has a nasty, almost maniacal and masochistic way of going on. To give you insight into what life was like for me, I carried a gym bag in my car containing extra clothes in the event that I experienced any "accidents". I had so many "loose bowel" episodes that I lost count. I could not even go for a walk at the park or somewhere just for fun without the fear of having another episode. I returned to work with all this going on plus I was also battling a serious lung infection at the same time which causes fatigue and chest discomfort. Daily rounds of heavy antibiotics for 2 years and the ever-present side effects of the medications which can also cause diarrhea and loose bowel. Auditing, even when you are healthy and strong, is tough, intimidating, demanding, and stressful which wear on you not only physically but also spiritually and emotionally.

Compounding my shaky health condition was my continuing difficulties with getting my rest at night. Since the tragic automobile accident in October 1981, I had a more and more difficult time going to sleep and staying asleep because of the neck, shoulder, and lower back injuries suffered in the accident. Proper sleep and rest was obviously essential for my healing and recovery from both prostate cancer and the lung infection. I was living in constant fear of suffering a relapse in my battle with cancer because I was still under a doctor's care, including my medical treatment for the lung infection. In late July 2011 I made the egregious mistake of taking Zanax along with Restoril or Temazepam to help me get my sleep. I began to experience hallucinations, hearing mysterious voices inside my head, delusions of seeing people that were not there, nightmares, and the dread I was being stalked by the police for whatever inexplicable reason. I became paranoid, looking out the windows because I believed I was being watched and under surveillance. I felt a sense of hopelessness and despair that made me feel like my life was coming to an end no matter what I tried to do. I even gave up both my dogs Misty and Buddy because of my deep depression and despair.

I eventually was admitted to Peachford Hospital on July 22, 2011 where I received much needed respite care and medical treatment. I stayed there at the hospital for 2 solid weeks and was prescribed the proper medication and treatment for depression and anxiety that I so desperately needed. Upon my return to the office, I applied for retirement from the State of Florida, effective September 30, 2012, and I haven't looked back. **Ephesians, Chapter 4, Verse 26 [New King James Version]**, states "**be angry, and do not sin. But <u>do not let the sun go down</u> on your wrath**".

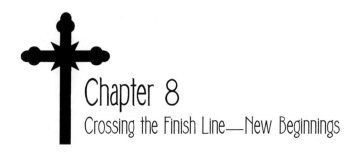

Chapter 8
Crossing the Finish Line—New Beginnings

Theodore Roosevelt was quoted as saying "[f]ar and away the best prize that life has to offer is the chance to work hard at work worth doing". Hard work has never killed anybody. Anything worthwhile always requires hard work, dedication, and perseverance. Never could I have imagined that when I started with the Florida Department of Revenue on October 1, 1984 as a lowly Tax Auditor I that this opportunity would be the last job I would ever have. I had been laid off from my accounting job at Arrow Aluminum in August 1984. Believe or not, my starting salary with the State of Florida was only $1,020 a month which was exactly the total monthly mortgage payments made for 2012 on the house my dad and I had bought in Roswell in December 2001. The fringe benefits included much needed health insurance coverage which I never had with Arrow Aluminum and a pension which today is almost extinct. However, if I had not been living with my parents in Sarasota at the time, I would not have been able to stay in Florida. Accounting job opportunities in the Sarasota County area that paid a decent salary were few and far between. My mother and father were always so proud of my accomplishments with the Department, but I owed my success to Jesse Poston who hired me, Marcia Sebestyen, and Colleen Forristall. They shared their vast tax knowledge and audit experience during the 5 years I was there in the Sarasota audit office. Pele, one of the greatest soccer players who ever lived, said **"[s]uccess is no accident. It is hard work, perseverance, learning, studying, sacrifice and most of all, love of what you are doing or learning to do."** I always felt that you know you have not worked hard enough on the job if you did not learn something new that day.

My horrific health history and my battle with depression during 2011 had not diminished my resolve to retire from the State of Florida. From what

I have read, mental illness and depression are no respecters of persons and know no barriers like race, creed, color, or nationality. Victims of its deadly grip include such famous and indomitable people as Winston Churchill, Abraham Lincoln, and professional basketball player Bill Walton.

Churchill suffered with depression when he was leading the British people to eventual victory during the terrible days of World War II. Lincoln also suffered with depression when he served as President during the bloody Civil War, the greatest moral, constitutional, and political crisis in this country's history. In doing so, Lincoln preserved the Union by abolishing slavery, strength-ening the federal government, and modernizing the nation's economy. Another remarkable fact about Lincoln's life is the obscure story about his birth. Thomas and Nancy Lincoln were expecting a child soon. Mr. Lincoln was made aware of the fact that the country doctor was not available because he had gone away on a long trip. He was the only doctor in this remote area where the Lincolns lived. One day a young woman came to their cabin and offered to be a midwife for delivery of the baby. The Lincolns were absolutely astonished and relieved that this young woman had appeared out of nowhere, but it was an answer to their prayers. When the baby was born, the Lincolns were so grateful for this woman's assistance in delivering the baby that they offered to pay her for her coming to their rescue to bring their son into the world. However, all she asked for from the Lincolns was to promise to name their son **Abraham**. And that they did. After the young woman had walked out the front door and left the cabin, Mr. Lincoln tried to catch up with her. When he walked outside the cabin and went out to the road, she was nowhere to be found. There was no way that she could have gone far. She had just vanished into thin air and was never seen again.

In the February 2016 issue of *ESPN Magazine*, the NBA's legendary center Bill Walton, who played for the equally legendary coach John Wooden at UCLA, talked candidly about how he had considered committing suicide when he was 56 because he could longer tolerate the debilitating nerve pain in his back. Walton has written a book entitled *Back From the Dead* where he reveals that he has undergone 37 operations on his back plus fusion surgeries on both ankles. He also talks about what chronic pain does to your psychological frame of mind by creating a dungeon of darkness, hopelessness, and depression. I can truly identify with what Walton is saying. I have been in that dungeon with the overwhelming feeling of no escape. I agree with Walton when he describes the 3 stages of suffering you are forced to endure: 1) you think you are facing the possibility of dying; 2) you wish you could die to end the suffering, and 3) you suddenly realize you have got to go on with your life and you are just stuck with the pain and discomfort, a hopeless feeling. My father's words echoed in what Walton said in the article. **Don't ever take your health for granted. Without it, you really do have nothing**.

The year 2012 was going to be a special period of time as I entered a new and exciting stage of my life. Retirement was a milestone I thought I would never achieve in my wildest dreams. It is so mind boggling that I had suffered with and have endured respiratory problems for over 5 decades plus all the other horrific health issues I have chronicled here, including life and death struggles. Mr. Walton, I have undergone **13 major surgeries** (3 lung operations, an emergency appendectomy, removal of my gall bladder, 2 seed implant surgeries for prostate cancer, 2 colon operations, 3 hernia repair surgeries, and dental implant surgery for TMJ) **plus over 20 surgical procedures on my lower back and hips** that were injured in the 1981 automobile accident. But I think you have me beat, Bill, with all of your surgeries.

Bo Jackson once said that **"[i]f my past didn't happen the way it did, I wouldn't be enjoying the present"**. My life certainly mirrors that statement. In November 2011, I made the fateful decision to put the house in Roswell up for sale. The sad memories of losing my father and my beloved dog Mischief, who both died in the house, still lingered there. I also felt very strongly that I needed a change of scenery and a fresh start somewhere else because I had suffered so much pain and heartache as well in the Roswell house. Unfortunately, for me the housing market in the Atlanta area was still reeling from the "Great Recession", and it was now a buyers' market. For 6 months I had no offers to buy the house, but I finally sold it in May 2012 after lowering the sales price considerably and taking a small loss. It was also very difficult for me to find another place to live because I was not financially prepared to buy another house at that time. As a result, I started looking for rental housing in the surrounding areas, and I luckily found an ideal size house to rent in Woodstock, Georgia. Before then, I had decided to retire early at age 62 on September 28, 2012 to fully enjoy outdoor activities, sports, the beach and the water, sailing, the mountains, working out at the gym, and hiking with my free time and also to do volunteer work such as serving at a soup kitchen and working in the church office. I have a passion for the outdoors and spend as much time as possible outside enjoying nature and the beauty of God's world. I always want to be near the water, if possible, because I enjoy boating and swimming. October 1, 2012 was my first day of retired life. My friends and family asked me what I was going to do with my free time. That was a good question. Here I was: it was 9:00AM in the morning, and I felt guilty. I had nothing planned and nowhere to go. I was so used to getting up at 5:00AM and battling traffic to get to the office on time. To me the saddest sound in the world is the alarm clock going off in the morning on a work day. I had to just plain slow down after working so hard and diligently as a tax auditor for 28 years. The negative job itself (always looking for taxpayer mistakes and assessing taxes due), hostile or uncooperative taxpayers who considered sales tax compliance a low priority, and the growing anti-government and anti-tax sentiment in the country had taken its toll on my psyche and overall health. I received a card congratulating me on my retirement. **The word "retirement" was spelled out in the card:**

> **R**elax and
> **E**njoy the ride
> **T**ry something new
> **I**magine the possibilities
> **R**emind yourself to play
> **E**xpect adventures
> **M**ake new plans
> **E**ntertain a few wild ideas
> **N**ap without guilt
> **T**ake time just for you

I grew up as an only child in the Atlanta area, and I am thankful for my Christian upbringing which has taught me to appreciate what I have and to treat others as I want them to treat me. I believe these qualities and Christian values are the result of my parents having survived the Depression years and being faithful to the church and God during their lifetimes. They taught me to trust in and serve the Lord each day with gratitude, and He will provide for us. I am a kind, caring, and compassionate person who also loves animals and dogs. I enjoy doing things for other people, especially those that are less fortunate than me. Benjamin Disraeli, who served Great Britain as its prime minister, once said "[a]ction may not always bring happiness; but there is no happiness without action."

In the quarterly devotional issue of *Christ in Our Home* for March 4, 2016, the author wrote about a popular ice cream parlor located in Howe, Indiana, with a storefront logo "Happiness Is Ice Cream". A sign on the parlor wall amplifies this message: **true happiness is found in Jesus Christ**. The Declaration of Independence proclaims the unalienable rights endowed by the Creator [God] Himself which include life, liberty, and the pursuit of happiness. We constantly are searching for peace and happiness in making a living, hard work and dedication resulting in success and good deeds, entertainment, leisure time, and family and friends. Our search for happiness pales in comparison to what is described in **Psalm 32, Verses 1-11** [New King James Version]:

> "**¹Blessed** *is he whose* **transgression** *is* **forgiven,**
> *Whose* **sin** *is* **covered.**
> **²Blessed** *is* **the man to whom the LORD does not impute**
> **iniquity,**
> **And in whose spirit** *there is* **no deceit.**
>
> **³When I kept silent, my bones grew old**
> **Through my groaning all the day long.**
> **⁴For day and night Your hand was heavy upon me;**
> **My vitality was turned into the drought of summer.** *Selah*
> **⁵I acknowledged my sin to You,**
> **And my iniquity I have not hidden.**
> **I said, "I will confess my transgressions to the LORD,"**
> **And You forgave the iniquity of my sin.** *Selah*
>
> **⁶For this cause everyone who is godly shall pray to You**
> **In a time when You may be found;**
> **Surely in a flood of great waters**
> **They shall not come near him.**

⁷ **You *are* my hiding place;**
You shall preserve me from trouble;
You shall surround me with songs of deliverance. *Selah*

⁸ **I will instruct you and teach you in the way you should go;**
I will guide you with My eye.
⁹ **Do not be like the horse *or* like the mule,**
***Which* have no understanding,**
Which must be harnessed with bit and bridle,
Else they will not come near you.

¹⁰ **Many sorrows *shall be* to the wicked;**
But he who trusts in the LORD, mercy shall surround him.
¹¹ **Be glad in the LORD and rejoice, you righteous;**
And shout for joy, all *you* upright in heart!"

The psalm gives a description of a heavenly happiness which is far deeper than any earthly joy. This happiness protects us even when we are in the darkest moments of life's journey like those I have faced and endured. We can only experience true peace, joy, and happiness when we accept the power and grace of God who surrounds us through the darkness and adversity life brings. Through Jesus Christ we also receive complete pardon from our sins and guilt.

For so long I wanted to do volunteer work at a food pantry or homeless shelter or serve the church in other capacities besides ushering and counting the offering. My job always stood in my way. According to Ronald Reagan, **"[w]e can't help everyone, but everyone can help someone."** Harry McBerry, my next-door neighbor in Woodstock, introduced me to Seniors Helping Seniors, and I met with Mary DuBois, the franchise owner, to discuss the nature and scope of their services and what the job entails. Seniors Helping Seniors was co-founded by Kiran Yocom who worked with Mother Teresa in India. **Mother Teresa proclaimed "[l]et no one ever come to you without leaving better and happier. Be the living expression of God's kindness: kindness in your face, kindness in your eyes, kindness in your smile."** Lucius Annaeus Seneca added that **"[w]herever there is a human being, there is an opportunity for a kindness."**

Seniors Helping Seniors provides non-medical services such as companion care, light housekeeping, cooking, grocery shopping, transportation to doctor's appointments, physical therapy, lab work, or other errands, house maintenance and minor repairs, yard work, and overnight 24-hour care. Julius Caesar stated that **"experience is the teacher of all things"**. I had life experience which I had derived from taking care of my dad for over 4 years. I joined Seniors Helping Seniors in December 2013, and I began my service for the organization on Valentine's Day in 2014. To say the least, it has been a humbling and rewarding experience for me.

As a caregiver, I have met some extraordinary people along the way that I would have not met otherwise. Gerald who was battling ALS [Lou Gehrig's Disease] and loved college basketball so much he knew all the teams and players; Chester, a World War II veteran and aircraft mechanic, who lived 95 years, married 66 years, and worked on the Apollo 11 space craft, part of which is still on the moon; Allen, who was in his 90's, attended West Point with legendary fellow cadets Glenn Davis and Doc Blanchard, and whose wife is a Hollywood actress; Frank, Floyd, and Chip who are valiantly battling Parkinson's; Allen whose wife is a member of the Kennedy family and who have a Yorkie mix named Scooter ["Scoots" for short] and is a "love sponge"; and Harold and Lee [short for Leroy] who are in the 90's and take no medication [both have a son, son-in-law, or grandson named David; my father's name was Harold Leroy].

Because of my parents, God's word has been my foundation, my staple for godly living, and my source of comfort, strength, and encouragement over the years since I left home to start a new life in Florida. The scriptures in **Colossians, Chapter 3 [New King James Version]** sum up my philosophy of service and a blueprint for my life:

> **"²² Servants, obey in all things your masters according to the flesh, not with eyeservice, as men-pleasers, but in sincerity of heart, fearing God. ²³ And whatever you do, do it heartily, as to the Lord and not to men, ²⁴ knowing that from the Lord you will receive the reward of the inheritance; for you serve the Lord Christ. ²⁵ But he who does wrong will be repaid for what he has done, and there is no partiality."**

I still must keep in mind that our works of service and our acts of generosity by themselves cannot save us as Paul explains in **Ephesians, Chapter 2, Verses 5 though 10 [New King James Version]:**

> **"5 even when we were dead in trespasses, made us alive together with Christ (by grace you have been saved), 6 and raised us up together, and made us sit together in the heavenly places in Christ Jesus, 7 that in the ages to come He might show the exceeding riches of His grace in His kindness toward us in Christ Jesus. 8 For by grace you have been saved through faith, and that not of yourselves; it isthe gift of God, 9 not of works, lest anyone should boast. 10 For we are His workmanship, created in Christ Jesus for good works, which God prepared beforehand that we should walk in them."**

I also learned about MUST Ministries from a friend. I had served in the food pantry at the Norcross Cooperative Ministry for a few months leading up to the diagnosis of prostate cancer in May 2010. As usual, my travel schedule with the Florida Department of Revenue played havoc with my availability to serve at the food pantry, and prostate cancer forced me to stop volunteering at the facility. MUST Ministries was founded in 1971 by Reverend Wayne Williams, and its initial programs included a grocery bus ministries for the elderly, a youth tutoring program, and outreach ministries for young people. With the help of more than 6,000 volunteers, MUST Ministries serves those in need in the Marietta, Smyrna, and Cherokee County communities. The organization provides emergency shelter, hot meals and groceries, clothing and shoes, supportive housing, summer lunch programs, Christmas toy shop, donation centers, and employment services, including job placement. In March 2013 I became involved as a volunteer serving in the kitchen and the dining room area of the Elizabeth Inn facility under the supervision of Lavon Minns and Red Pratt. I help unload donations of food by the surrounding community, answer the telephone when necessary, help set up the dining room area to serve lunch to the homeless, scan cards that track and account for all those that are eating at the Elizabeth Inn that particular day, take out the trash, mop floors, and help clean up the parking lot area.

After all is said and done, I still had unfinished business with strengthening my lower back and neck. I never gave up hope on finding the correct set of exercises and proper workout techniques to strengthen my core muscles in my abdominal area, hips, and lower back. Over the years doctors, chiropractors, physical therapists, surgeons, and osteopaths had given me several exercises to do, but none of them were effective in easing my pain and discomfort and strengthening my lower extremities as well. I always knew exercise, proper diet, and rest were vital to my overall health. Much to my dismay, I had to stop running on January 29, 1988. Running was just jarring my lower back and hips so badly I could no longer tolerate the pain. My quality of life was almost nonexistent without running because it kept my lungs and respiratory tract functioning properly. Through several discussions with many health care professionals, I was told that walking was beneficial, but walking is just not the same as running or jogging. Nevertheless, I started to dream about jogging again, feeling that adjusting my stride and slowing my pace to a military shuffle would alleviate the jarring of my lower back causing my pain and discomfort in running. I had to consider alternatives to jogging, so I eventually worked out on the treadmill, an exercise bike with a large seat, and a rowing machine at the YMCA.

In March 2013 I received a flyer in the mail from Gold's Gym in Woodstock, and I eventually joined the gym after I had been working out for awhile at the YMCA in Canton 15 miles away. God had planted the seed for yet another miracle. It was a decision which has transformed my life and began the odyssey I am still embarked upon to this day. I had not had any massage therapy or chiropractic manipulations for quite some time because of the cost. On July 10, 2013 I went to see Dr. Jonathan Snow with **Peak Performance Chiropractic**. I had noticed a banner on the 2nd floor balcony of Gold's Gym that informed members about **Peak Performance Chiropractic**. I discussed my health history and the nature and cause of the injuries suffered in the tragic automobile accident in October 1981 with Dr. Snow. According to his Internet website peakperformancewoodstock.com, "Dr. Snow is a Board Certified Chiropractic Sports Physician® and a member of the American Chiropractic Board of Sports Physicians™. He graduated from Logan College of Chiropractic in St. Louis, Missouri in 2006, and later had the unique opportunity to receive post-graduate sports medicine training at the Olympic Training Center in Colorado Springs, Colorado. Dr.

Snow also holds a bachelor's degree in Exercise Science from Brigham Young University. **He specializes in treating athletic injuries, providing non-surgical strategies for pain management, and developing customized exercise plans to correct chronic stress and muscular disorders.** Dr. Snow is one of only 35 Certified Chiropractic Sports Physicians® in Georgia, and he is the only certified sports chiropractor in Woodstock. Through his expertise in the field of sports medicine, Dr. Snow has had the distinction of serving as a team chiropractor for a number of professional and Division I collegiate teams and athletes, and has helped countless recreational athletes, runners, and weightlifters improve their performance and enjoyment in their respective endeavors. Dr. Snow is passionate about helping active individuals and athletes return to full activity when sidelined by injury or nagging pain. **He offers patients classic chiropractic techniques with a modern sports medicine perspective, and utilizes hands-on adjusting, neuromuscular therapy, taping, and exercise to address muscular and joint dysfunction."**

His approach for medical treatment and physical therapy was exactly what I needed to connect the dots, beginning with the neuromuscular massage therapy performed by David Shue and then the prolotherapy surgical procedures performed by Dr. Marvin Hodson, Dr. David Kudelko, and Dr. Ken Knott. **Dr. Snow focuses upon 3 areas of physical therapy for the treatment of both my neck and lower back: flexibility, stability, and mobility. <u>It is hard to comprehend that I had waited almost 32 years for someone to give me a set of exercises to heal and strengthen my back.</u>** Dr. Snow was right under my nose at Gold's Gym in Woodstock. **I had once told my father that if I had a year or two off from work, I could make a comeback you can tell your grandkids about. Retirement afforded me the opportunity to do just that.**

The 4 keys to healthy living and long life are:

1. **Live a godly life (Matthew, Chapter 6, Verse 33, says ....seek ye first the kingdom of God and His righteousness therein, and all these things you need will be given unto you.)**
2. **Eating right and taking vitamin supplements.**
3. **Getting plenty of sleep and rest.**
4. **Regular exercise.**

I also have tried to abide by God's Word in **Matthew, Chapter 6 [New King James Version]**:

"¹⁹**Do not lay up for yourselves treasures on earth, where moth and rust destroy and where thieves break in and steal; ²⁰but lay up for yourselves treasures in heaven, where neither moth nor rust destroys and where thieves do not break in and steal. ²¹For where your treasure is, there your heart will be also. ²²The lamp of the body is the eye. If therefore your eye is good, your whole body will be full of light. ²³But if your eye is bad, your whole body will be full of darkness. If therefore the light that is in you is darkness, how great *is* that darkness! ²⁴No one can serve two masters; for either he will hate the one and love the other, or else he will be loyal to the one and despise the other. You cannot serve God and mammon.**"

Amazingly in the spring of 2014 I played softball again for the first time since September 1982. I never thought I would ever play the game I loved so much again. I played on 2 championship softball teams in 2014 and 1championship softball team during 2015. I cried for joy when I had stepped onto the softball field for the first time in 32 years. I even began to ride a shiny bright red Del Rio bicycle that I decided to buy in 2015. I felt like a little kid again. I guess I am now living my "second" childhood or maybe my "second adulthood".

I now have 2 Schnauzers which I rescued after my beloved Misty passed away on January 10, 2015. I adopted a pure white male Schnauzer 2 weeks later from **Schnauzer Love Rescue**, a non-profit rescue organization of volunteers which is devoted to finding homes for all abandoned and unwanted Miniature Schnauzers through the "Family Match Program". The organization also helps find a home for those dogs whose families had to give up their pets. I named him Spunky because of his high energy, headstrong personality, and playful nature. Later in December 2015 I adopted a purebred black male Schnauzer named Harry who was rescued from an animal shelter by Lucky Day Rescue, Inc. Harry is exactly the opposite of Spunky—calm, mild-mannered, and easy-going around people (a "love sponge"). Salt and pepper I call them. Great blessings from God!

During a stirring speech in November 1942, Winston Churchill addressed his embattled countrymen in Great Britain during World War II and proclaimed "[n]ow this is not the end. It is not even the beginning of the end. But it is, perhaps, the end of the beginning". It is not how you start the race of life, but how you finish it. William James wrote to "act as if what you do makes a difference. It does". My plan for retirement was a simple one: **Keep on living, keep on giving! Life is too short not to.**